Your Gift

I wanted to show my appreciation that you support my work so
I've put together a free gift for you.

http://bonusfreebook.org/

Just visit the link above to download it now.

I know you will love this gift.

If you like this book, you can see and buy my other books on this
link:

https://www.amazon.com/Lisa-
Brook/e/B079TZXP62/ref=sr_ntt_srch_lnk_4?qid=1518768684&sr=1-
4

Thank you for attention!

With love,

Lisa Brook

TABLE OF CONTENTS

INTRODUCTION

Meal preppers, welcome! This book is all about meal prepping, from tips and tricks, benefits and secrets, all the way to the recipes for breakfast, lunch, and dinner. If you have a goal of losing weight and trimming down your waist, you've started at the right place as meal prepping can really help you to reach your slimming objectives. There's something about being organized and dedicated which makes you really want to stick to your goals and eat the foods you know will deliver you to your healthiest weight yet.

These recipes are not "diet" recipes; they are healthy, nutritious, filling, and tasty recipes. I don't believe you need to cut out any food groups or deprive yourself of something in order to lose weight. In fact, eating properly, eating enough, and eating foods that satisfy you, will result in weight-loss you can maintain and sustain. So, if you're looking for a particular diet or eating style, then this might not be the book for you! But I hope it is, as I know you'll love these recipes as much as I do.

Oh, I should add a bit about me! I am not a nutritionist or dietitian. But I am someone who has successfully lost weight through sensible and healthy eating, and of course, meal prepping! I want to pass on my recipes and my knowledge of meal prepping so you too can experience the same success and health benefits.

Please consult your doctor or nutritionist for advice and guidance if you are looking to lose large amounts of weight, or if you have health issues which might be affected due to a change in your diet. This book is a friendly and supportive guideline to help you lose weight in a healthy way, without extreme changes or deprivation.

Now, let's get into the ins and outs of meal prepping!

CHAPTER I: WHAT IS MEAL PREPPING?

Meal prepping is the art of preparing your meals the night (or a few nights) before actually eating them. It usually involves preparing a few portions of each meal, packing them away in airtight containers, and storing in the fridge. Many people prep their meals these days, because it saves time, encourages healthy eating, and controls portions. Sometimes, the meal is completely prepared and cooked in its entirety before being stacked away in the fridge or freezer until it is needed. Whereas sometimes, meals are only partially prepared so they can be cooked right before eating. For example, you can prep lasagna by cooking the sauces and layering it all up before covering and storing in the fridge, raw. You would then place the lasagna into a preheated oven before eating the next night. Whatever prepping method you choose, it's a great way to manage your time and your diet!

CHAPTER II: WHY MEAL PREP?

There are countless reasons to get into the joys of meal prepping, but here are some of the top reasons:

SAVES TIME

By setting aside a chunk of time to get all or most of your meals for the week prepped, you are saving yourself hours of frazzled and rushed cooking throughout the coming days. You can wake up in the morning, grab your prepped breakfast from the fridge, throw your prepped lunch into your bag (ready to eat as soon as you're ready!), and come home to a ready-made dinner you only need to heat in the oven or microwave. Not only you save your precious time on cooking, you also save thinking time. I don't know about you, but thinking about what to have for breakfast, lunch and dinner always takes up far more of my time than it should!

SAVES MONEY

When you decide what to eat for lunch and dinner as you go through the week, you end up heading to the supermarket every couple of days, which increases your chance of spending money on things you don't really need. But when you make a plan of what you will eat for each meal throughout the entire week, you can do one shopping spree where you would buy only what you need for those particular meals. You will end up with far less unnecessary items, and more money in your wallet!

KEEPS YOU HEALTHY WITH PORTION CONTROL AND PLANNING

Meal prepping is all about packing away single servings of food for each meal. Therefore, you only make enough for a certain number of portions, with no leftovers. I'm sure you can sympathize with me when I say that leftovers are my absolute downfall! When I don't prep my meals, I end up eating far larger portions than I actually need, because it's right there in front of me! When you get to eat your breakfast, lunch and dinner, all you have to eat is the single portion you have made, nothing more.

Of course, this does mean you need to prepare sensible portion sizes in the first place, which I have aimed to provide in these recipes. You can adjust the ingredient quantities to suit your personal portion-size preference for your BMI, calorie requirements and activity levels.

HELPS YOU TO REACH YOUR GOALS

Quite simply, prepping your meals helps you to remain in control of your eating habits in order to reach your weight-loss and health-related goals. You can assess the calories and macros for each recipe and make sure they fit with your weight-loss eating plan, so you know that each meal you enjoy is going to help you get to where you want to be.

This works two ways! One: the actual meal-prepping process gives you some time for yourself to quietly potter away and enjoy being in the kitchen, with busy hands and lots of creating to do. Two: you will have so much more time for yourself (and for your loved ones) throughout the week than when you would usually be rushing around trying to prepare meals from a scratch.

CHAPTER III: TIPS AND TRICKS

Trying to think of things to have for each meal can be tiresome and draining, so it's great to have a compilation of your favorite dishes, and some new ones to try too! When you come across a dish you really love and you would like it to be a regular in your rotation, print or write it out and stick it in your own homemade recipe book! Hopefully you'll find some new favorites in this book to add to your cooking repertoire too.

If you like to freestyle some of your meals and forgo the use of a recipe, make sure you write down the ingredients you used and a rough rundown of the method, so you can recreate it another time! You'll end up with your very own, self-curated recipe book.

GET YOUR PARTNER OR FAMILY IN ON THE MEAL-PREP FUN

If you're prepping for a partner or for your family as well as for yourself, don't take on all the work! Get your family or loved one involved, and treat it as a chance for some quality time for talking and laughing as you prep your meals. If you have kids, give them an easy job so they can practice their food-prep skills while making them feel useful and appreciated in the kitchen with Mom or Dad. This will help to establish the meal-prep time as a fun and relaxing thing to do, which means you'll be far more likely to keep the routine up!

MAKE A DEDICATED MEAL-PREP BOX TO KEEP IN THE PANTRY

In my pantry, you will find a large box filled with containers, measuring cups and spoons, and a range of regularly-used ingredients. I keep oats, nuts, seeds, canned goods such as beans and corn, olive oil, salt, pepper, herbs, spices, and more. When I embark on each meal-prep session I place this box on the counter and it has all of the essentials I need to create many meals. All I need to do is get my fresh produce, meat and dairy from the fridge and I'm good to go. This makes life quicker and easier as it means you don't need to rummage around in cupboards, shelves, and drawers to find utensils, containers, and ingredients.

CHOOSE A MEAL-PREP DAY AND MAKE SURE IT'S A RELAXING EXPERIENCE

If you plan your meal prepping days right, you will begin to really look forward to each meal prep session. It shouldn't be a stressful, rushed, or cumbersome activity, so choose a day when you've got a large chunk of time all to yourself. I believe that Sunday afternoons and evenings are the best, as there are rarely social or work activities on Sunday evenings (and there should never be!). I usually start at 2pm and just meander through the process for as long as it takes and I feel it really does help me to relax. I usually put a podcast or movie on my computer and watch or listen to it as I quietly work – it's a great time to binge watch a great show! The great thing about Sunday is that you wake up on Monday morning with all of your meals planned and prepped. Choose a day and time that works best for you and do whatever you can to make the experience enjoyable. You could even invite a friend or two around to chatter away with you as you prep (perhaps with a nice glass of wine while you're at it?).

CHAPTER IV: 9 RULES FOR SUCCESSFUL MEAL PREPPING

KEEP IT SIMPLE

Start with some simple recipes with minimal ingredients. Most of the recipes in this book are simple and easy to make, without many fancy ingredients or tricky steps. Don't overwhelm yourself by prepping complicated or fiddly dishes – keep it simple until you feel confident to branch out. This will save you time and money, and it will make your first prepping experiences easy and enjoyable.

UTILIZE THE FREEZER

Frozen prepped meals are a lifesaver during busy and chaotic times. A good way to utilize the freezer is to double the recipe for a particular meal and put a half of the servings in the fridge for the consequent days, and put the other half in the freezer for later down the track. You'll be very pleased you did so, especially during the times when your meal-prep game schedule is slipping!

KEEP YOUR MACROS IN MIND: PROTEINS, CARBS, FATS

You don't want to sit down to your prepped lunch only to find that it's too filling or not filling enough due to the unbalanced nutritional value. Remember to include a portion of protein, some good fats, and some healthy wholegrain carbs for optimum energy and satiety. Most of the recipes in this book have a great balance of macros, but you can adjust them to suit your needs and preferences.

STOCK-UP ON FLAVOR-PACKING NON-PERISHABLES

Herbs, spices, vinegars, oils, and natural flavorings can turn any simple dish into a tasty masterpiece, with very few added calories. What's more, they last for a very long time in the pantry so you don't need to worry about using them up before their best-before date. Splash out on a big haul of natural, flavor-giving ingredients to pack into your meal-prep box. This means that you can use simple-base ingredients, and then adjust the flavors with the addition of healthy and low-cal seasonings.

INVEST IN STORAGE EQUIPMENT

This is an important one. To successfully prep, you need containers to store your meals in. High-quality plastic or glass containers with airtight lids are ideal, especially if you can find a set which includes different sizes. Small, single-serve containers are really handy for breakfasts such as oats and chia pudding, and snacks such as fruit and nut mix. Pyrex bowls which have airtight lids are perfect for large salads and soups. Have a shop around and find yourself a few value packs, and allocate a special box, drawer, or cupboard, especially for your meal-prep containers.

GET CREATIVE WITH COLOR

During my own meal prepping journey I found that using bright and varied colors really helped me to get excited about making, and eating my prepped meals. A pile of red cabbage with bright red bell peppers and some vibrant green cilantro – beautiful! Rich yellow corn kernels, inky black beans, glossy red chili, and pale green avocado looks as amazing as it tastes. If you're like me, then you'll get a kick out of putting together beautiful and fresh-looking meals to fill your containers. Fresh fruits, veggies, herbs, and rich spices are the best sources of edible colors.

PREDICT YOUR CRAVINGS AND PREP ACCORDINGLY

If you don't feel like eating a particular meal, then don't prep it. Don't think that you must eat a certain type of dish simply because it seems like the healthiest option. You can make any dish healthy! Even if it's traditionally considered a junk food. For example, you will find recipes for burgers and rich pastas in this book, but they are the nutritious versions which fit in with your weight-loss plans. If you've got a craving for sweeter dishes, then try some yummy oatmeal with dates for breakfast! If you feel like something a bit heavier for dinner (tiredness, hormones, and overindulgence can make us crave for comfort foods) then choose a recipe for dinner with sweet potatoes and beans to fill you up. The bottom line? Prep foods you want to eat that particular week! This way, you'll avoid seeking other foods or snacks to satisfy you in between the meals.

MAKE A PLAN AND STICK TO IT

This is where you need to be a bit strict and structured. Decide on a day to complete your prepping, set the time aside, and stick to it. Get your grocery shopping done on the same day so your foods and meats are fresh, then set aside a couple of hours to prep, prep, prep! If you end up missing a prep day and you don't have the time to make up for it, you might find yourself slip back into day-to-day meals and the unhealthy choices and unbalanced portion sizes may creep back. Once the routine has been established it will be so easy!

KEEP IT FUN

Cooking should be as fun as eating, in my opinion! And the same goes for prepping. If you enjoy yourself, you'll get into a positive mindset about the meal prepping, and a positive mindset about the food that will follow on.

There are many ways to make the meal-prep sessions fun! Play music, have a glass of wine, watch your favorite TV show, anything that relaxes you and puts you at ease as you work. Weight loss needn't be a drag, it can actually be an enjoyable and nourishing experience if you make the process work in a way that you enjoy.

CHAPTER V: HOW TO MEAL PREP LIKE A PRO

You will get into your own meal-prep rhythm, but here is a step-by-step guide to meal prepping like a pro which you can use as a guide when you first get started.

SCHEDULE YOUR PREP DAY

Take a look at your diary or calendar (or an app on your phone you use to schedule your days!) and find a day when you can set aside a good 3 hours for meal prepping. Weekends are ideal, especially Sundays, so you can prep for the entire week coming. Set the time aside for meal planning, shopping, and prepping. Don't double-book yourself; treat it like an important appointment you must keep.

WRITE YOUR MEAL PLAN

Sit down with a pad and paper and write down what you want to eat for breakfast, lunch, and dinner throughout the coming week. Try to keep it to 2 variations per week. For example: 2 different options for breakfast, lunch and dinner, as opposed to a different meal every day, or the same thing every day.

Compose a shopping list based on your meal plan, taking into account the items you already have in your kitchen.

GO SHOPPING

Head to the supermarket and strictly follow your shopping list! Don't be tempted to stray and buy items you don't need. When you get home, unpack your groceries and place them in the easy-to-find places, or even leave them on the table if you're going to start prepping immediately. Remember to refrigerate meats and dairy. If you have a "prep box", put your dried or nonperishable goods into it so they're ready to go for prepping.

PREPPING

First, figure out which steps you can multi-task. If you need to cook something in the oven, prepare to get another task done as it cooks. If you need to let something soak or cool, use that time to complete other steps. Figure out which meals are the most time-consuming and get started with those first, using these little bits of spare time in the process to complete quicker tasks such as mixing granola or slicing fresh veggies.

PACK, LABEL AND STORE

Before you begin, it's a good idea to clear a shelf in your fridge (and freezer, if using) so you don't have to shuffle things around and pack things into awkward places when it comes to storing your freshly-prepared meals.

Use the most compact containers you can when storing your meals. This is when having a range of different sizes will come in very handy!

If you like, you can label your containers by sticking a removable, plain sticker onto the lid and marking it with a marker. Write down the date you cooked/prepped the meal so you know how long it has been in the fridge. This will help you to ensure your meals are always fresh.

Pack away your prepped meals, clean up, sit back, and relax!

CHAPTER VI: WEIGHT LOSS – NUTRITION, CALORIES, MACROS AND MICROS

HOW WEIGHT LOSS WORKS – WITH A PERSONAL STORY TO MATCH!

This will have to be a simplified version of the weight loss process! And keep in mind, not everyone is the same and some people lose the weight more easily than others, and others may keep weight on for various health reasons. Make sure you see your doctor first if you are aiming to lose weight, as they can look through your medical history and point out any potential patterns or issues, which could help you find the best method for you. Now that that's out of the way, we can get into the general rules and sciences behind the weight loss.

So, when you eat food, you are taking in energy (calories). When you move and exercise, you are burning calories. When you burn more calories than the amount you have consumed, you will lose weight. Keep in mind that your body needs a basic number of calories in order to survive and keep your organs running, which is why it's very important to eat enough. I highlight this because when I first started to consider calories I was a bit taken aback by the notion of "burning more calories than you take in", thinking I would have to burn 1800 calories worth of exercise a day! But perhaps that was just my very silly mistake; you are probably a lot more intelligent than that!

When you reach a calorie deficit, your body begins to turn to energy sources, which are already stored in your body, i.e. the stored fat. Sometimes, muscle can also be used for energy, which does result in weight loss, but it also results in muscle loss and a less-toned physique. You can remedy this by incorporating strength training into your fitness routine, as well as the high intensity cardio. By doing this, you are helping your body to burn fat as well as build muscle at the same time. You also need to eat properly to give your body enough protein and energy to get through those workouts and repair those muscles properly afterwards!

Some people opt for the low-calorie method of weight loss, and I have also tried that. It worked for a while but I couldn't sustain it, so I had to turn to another method. I decided to ramp-up my workouts and eat a more well-rounded diet, full of nutritious foods, and enough of them. By training with weights and high intensity cardio, my metabolism became faster and more efficient, and my increased muscle mass helped me burn more calories.

CALORIES

"Calories" is basically another word for energy. When you eat, you are consuming energy, which your body uses to function and grow. If you eat too many calories, you will put on extra weight; if you reduce them, you will lose weight. You can figure out how many calories you need in order to lose weight by punching your weight, height, age, gender, and activity level into an online calorie-counter. It will tell you how many calories you need to consume in order to lose, gain or maintain weight. A good rule of thumb is to reduce your calorific intake by 300-500 calories. This can be done pretty easily just by cutting out high-calorie foods such as processed treats, cakes, ice cream, white starches and alcohol.

MACRONUTRIENTS

Macronutrients are the main groups your food is categorized under: carbs, fats, and proteins. Each of these has a particular function in the body, and they are all important for weight-loss and general health. I know there are many people out there who banish carbs, but let's make this book a carb-friendly zone!

CARBOHYDRATES

Carbs give you energy! Your body adores carbs because it's an easy energy source. Carbohydrates, especially those found in starchy or sugary foods are often very high in calories, which is why people avoid overeating carbs when trying to manage their weight. When you don't burn off the energy you consume, your body stores it as fat – so it's best to eat a high-carb meal on days when you are active and exercising. As long as you get the carbs from the whole, natural sources with slow-releasing energy, there's absolutely no need to fear them! Do you want to eat bread? Opt for a wholegrain sourdough from a real bakery as opposed to a white loaf from the supermarket (these are often full of sugar and refined white flour). Are you feeling like pasta? Opt for a whole-white or gluten-free variety and take note of the serving size on the packet and stick to it so you don't add extra calories with large portions.

Carbs to eat:

- Starchy veggies such as sweet potatoes
- Fruits and berries
- Whole-grains such as quinoa, brown rice, oats

- Wholegrain breads and pastas

- Processed, white flour (cakes and baked goods, white bread)
- White pasta
- White rice (in moderation is fine, but brown rice is far better)
- Sugary foods (sweets, cakes, ice cream…all of the classic sugary snacks!)

FATS

Healthy fats are important for the body to function properly. Fats make you feel satiated and full, and they help the body to absorb and process essential nutrients and proteins. Good fats found in foods such as fish and avocadoes are great for cognitive (brain) health and keeping the skin in good condition. Adding a source of healthy fat to your dinner will help you to feel satisfied. Opt for nuts, seeds, avocado, fish and olive oil.

Fatty foods to eat:

- Avocadoes
- Nuts and seeds
- Olive oil
- Oily fish such as salmon and tuna

Fatty foods to avoid:

- Fried foods (fast foods)
- Processed fats such as margarine

PROTEINS

Protein is very important for muscle growth, that's why hard-core power-lifters are always guzzling protein shakes and egg whites! If we didn't eat any protein, our cells, bones, muscles, nails, (basically our whole body!) couldn't repair and renew itself and grow stronger. It's important to incorporate proteins into your diet so your body can remain strong and supported. Protein is also very satiating so it fills you up and keeps cravings at bay.

Protein to eat:

- Eggs
- Lean red meat
- Lean chicken
- Fish
- Unsweetened yogurt
- Beans and lentils
- Tofu

- Fatty meats

MICRONUTRIENTS

Micronutrients are far more commonly-known as vitamins and minerals. We usually take supplements and pills to boost our micronutrient levels, especially in the winter when we are prone to sicknesses and viruses. However, you really can get enough micronutrients through a proper diet (unless you have a condition which hinders your body's ability to absorb and hold onto certain micronutrients). As long as you eat lots of fresh fruits, veggies, lean meats, grains and seeds you should be getting enough micronutrients. However, blood tests can detect micronutrient deficiencies and you can take supplements to remedy this.

Here are the important micronutrients to keep an eye out for:

- Iron
- Magnesium
- Folate
- Calcium
- Zinc
- B, A, C and E vitamins

CHAPTER VII: GROCERY LIST – SIMPLE, ACCESSIBLE, AND AFFORDABLE INGREDIENTS

This grocery list is a rough guide to healthy shopping and these ingredients are all featured in the recipes for breakfast, lunch and dinner. Please feel free to adjust the list according to what's in season, especially when it comes to fresh produce.

I haven't added quantities for you, because you may be feeding one person, or you may be feeding many! So simply plan your meals for the week, figure out how many portions you will be making, and choose your quantities accordingly.

Happy shopping!

- Broccoli
- Spinach
- Carrots
- Kale
- Onions
- Garlic
- Bananas
- Zucchini
- Swiss chard
- Bell peppers (all colors)
- Green onions (scallions)

- Frozen mixed berries
- Frozen green beans

- Free range eggs
- Whole milk
- Feta cheese
- Ricotta cheese
- Cheddar cheese

- Chicken thighs

- Chicken breasts
- Lean beef steak
- Lean lamb leg steak
- Smoked salmon
- Fresh white fish fillets

- Wholegrain pasta
- Wholegrain or sourdough bread
- Wholegrain wraps
- Wholegrain pita breads

GRAINS:

- Quinoa
- Wholegrain rolled oats
- Brown rice
- Couscous

NUTS, SEEDS AND DRIED FRUITS:

- Whole raw almonds
- Whole raw walnuts
- Pumpkin seeds
- Sunflower seeds
- Chia seeds
- Flaxseeds
- Dates
- Prunes
- Raisins
- Dried apricots
- Desiccated or threaded coconut
- Nori sheets (seaweed)

OILS, SAUCES, VINEGARS:

- Olive oil
- Coconut oil
- Apple cider vinegar
- Balsamic vinegar
- Sesame oil
- Soy sauce
- Lamb broth
- Chicken broth

- Beef broth

<u>*CANNED GOODS:*</u>

- Black beans
- Kidney beans
- Corn kernels
- Canned chopped tomatoes
- Coconut milk
- Canned lentils

CHAPTER VIII: MEAL PREP RECIPES

ABOUT THESE RECIPES

When reading the shopping list, you might have noticed these recipes do not cut out any food groups. I don't believe you have to cut carbs or fats in order to lose weight! As long as you are active and you are eating fresh, whole food and remaining mindful of portion sizes, you can eat the foods you love. One thing these recipes do not contain is refined sugar. Fruits and the odd drizzle of honey may make an appearance, but none of the processed stuff!

SERVES

Each recipe states how many servings it makes. If you are prepping your meals only for yourself, then you will have as many servings as the recipe makes. But if you are cooking for two, then you will have half, and your partner will have the other half. Therefore, keep in mind how many days you want a particular recipe to last for, and adjust the quantities accordingly. For example, if you want Bircher muesli every day for 6 days for yourself, then add an extra half of the ingredient list on top of the indicated amounts to make 6 servings (the recipe makes 4). I haven't made each recipe cater to a whole week because not all the recipes are great enough after a few days in the fridge, but that's up to you!

CONTAINERS

Containers are KEY when it comes to meal prepping. I have indicated which kind of containers you will need to store each prepped recipe. Most of them are pretty flexible and a normal bowl covered with a cling wrap is completely fine. However, if you're planning to take your prepped meals (especially lunches) to work, then airtight containers with reliable lids are the best. Look for some bargains and get a few value packs of containers!

TIME

This simply refers to the amount of time it will take you to complete the preparation, including any cooking if required. It does not include overnight chilling time. These times are approximate, as everyone preps at a different pace!

INGREDIENTS

Just as it sounds, this is where you find all of the ingredients you will need to make your prepped meal. I haven't added salt or pepper to the ingredients lists as I'm certain you will have those ingredients at the ready at all times.

DIRECTIONS

I have aimed to provide clear and precise directions so you can get your meal prepping done quickly, without having to guess or decipher any missing steps.

NUTRITIONAL VALUE

Here you will find the approximate calorie count, and the fat, protein and carbohydrate content in grams for each serving. I have used My Fitness Pal to gather this information, which is a very accurate source. However, I might use different brands of certain foods which might alter the nutritional content slightly, so please take these numbers as approximate and not exact.

BREAKFAST

I believe in eating a filling, energy-rich breakfast every day, especially when trying to lose weight. Many of these recipes contain wholegrain rolled oats, which I consider to be a Holy Grail ingredient! The carbohydrate content in most of these recipes is pretty high, because I think it's best to consume the majority of your carbs in the first half of the day for your energy needs. There is a mixture of sweet and savory, hot and cold recipes to choose from.

BIRCHER MUESLI WITH APPLE AND CINNAMON

The recipe includes oats and grated apple soaked in yoghurt and milk overnight, with a dash of warming cinnamon. This is a very simplified recipe, as I find that a less "busy" bircher in the morning is the best. However, you can add extra nuts and seeds if you wish, just remember that it will change the nutritional value.

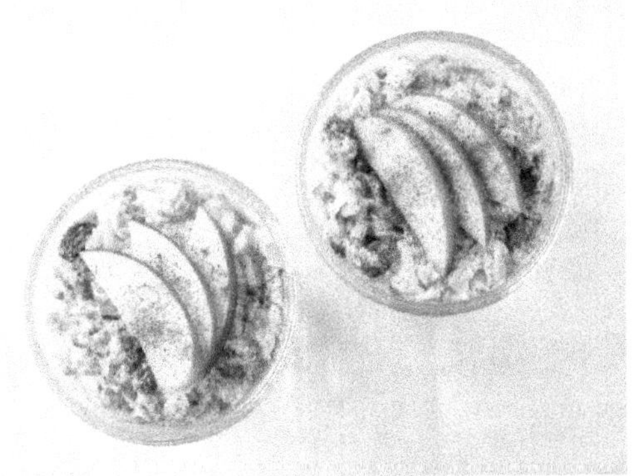

Serves: 4 prepped servings

Container: 4 small containers or small bowls or ramekins

Time: approximately 10 minutes

Nutritional info per serving:

- Calories: 185
- Fat: 3 grams
- Protein: 4 grams
- Carbs: 33 grams

Ingredients:

- 1 ½ cups wholegrain rolled oats
- 2 apples, skin on, grated
- 1 tsp. ground cinnamon
- 1 cup almond milk (or any other milk you prefer)
- 1 cup plain, unsweetened yogurt

Method:

1. Place the oats, grated apple, cinnamon, milk, and yogurt into a bowl and stir to combine. The mixture should be wet and reasonably thick, but it will depend on the brand of yogurt you are using. If your mixture seems a bit too dry or too thick, add a bit more milk or even some water if you don't want to change the calorie count.

2. Divide the mixture between your four containers or bowls, cover, and place in the fridge.

3. In the morning, simply grab it from the fridge and enjoy! You'll love this cold, filling, and refreshing breakfast.

TROPICAL SMOOTHIE IN FREEZER PACKETS

Smoothies in freezer packets are lifesavers! These ones are full of tropical ingredients for a fresh and naturally sweet morning smoothie. Simply add water or milk, blitz, and drink. Easy! Note: adding milk will adjust the nutritional info as the value provided is for the contents of the smoothie packet only.

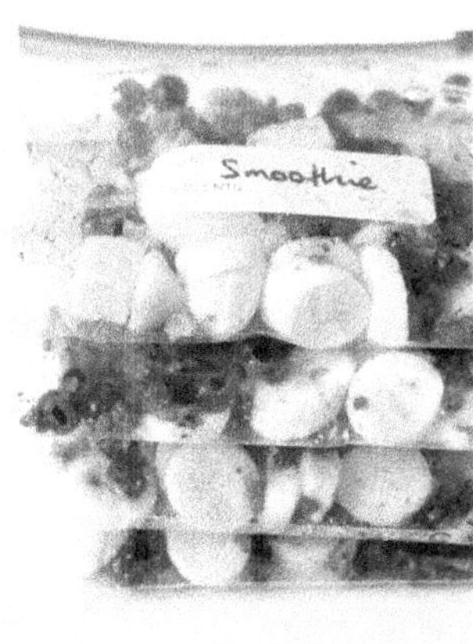

Serves: 7 freezer packets (one smoothie per packet)

Container: 7 small sealable, freezer-friendly bags

Time: approximately 10 minutes

Nutritional info per serving – with water added only:

- Calories: 145
- Fat: 1 gram
- Protein: 3 grams
- Carbs: 36 grams

Ingredients:

- 3 bananas, peeled and chopped into chunks
- 2 fresh mangoes, peeled, flesh cut into chunks
- 3 cups frozen or fresh mixed berries
- 2 cups chopped kale

Method:

1. Place the banana, mango, berries, and kale into a bowl and stir to combine.
2. Divide the mixture into your 7 freezer-safe bags, seal, and place in the freezer.
3. In the morning, simply throw the contents of one freezer smoothie packet into your blender, add a cup of water or milk (coconut milk

would be great with this recipe!) and blend. For some extra
sustenance, you could add a handful of oats and some yogurt.

As boring as this "recipe" may sound, boiled eggs are a meal-prepper's dream. A boiled egg is a great "side dish" to any breakfast, as they provide a great dose of protein. A boiled egg and a prepped smoothie for breakfast? Yes please.

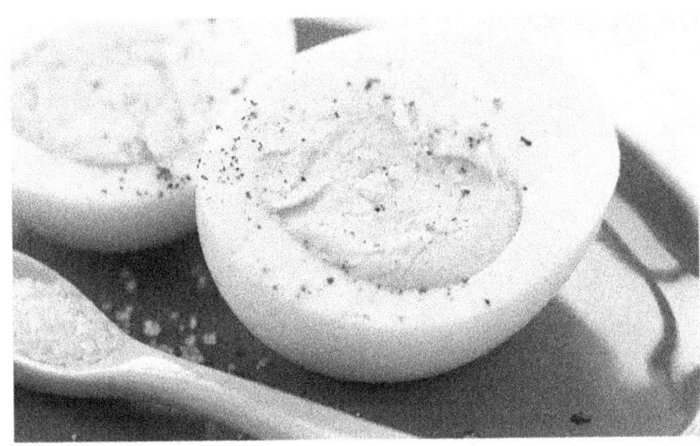

Serves: 7 boiled eggs (one egg per serving, as a protein hit)

Container: you can store these any way you like, you could even put them in the egg holder inside your fridge to save using a separate bowl or container

Time: approximately 20 minutes (including cooling time)

Nutritional info per serving:

- Calories: 70
- Fat: 5 grams
- Protein: 6 grams
- Carbs: 0 grams

Ingredients:

- 7 eggs

Method:

1. Bring a small pot of water to a boil (enough water to thoroughly cover the eggs).
2. Turn the heat down to low so the boiling is not so vigorous.
3. Very carefully place the eggs into the pot using a large spoon.
4. Set the timer to 9 minutes and leave the eggs in the boiling water.
5. Once the timer beeps, place the pot under a tap of cold water until all of the water in the pot is cold.
6. Leave the eggs to cool in the cold water for about 10 minutes before placing them in the fridge.
7. I leave the shell on my hard-boiled eggs until right before eating them, as I find it easier to store them with the shell on.

FRUIT SALAD WITH LEMON AND HONEY

Look, I know many people would say that eating lots of fruit (and added honey!) is not "healthy" for weight-loss due to the sugar content. However, these are the natural sugars, and these fruits also provide lots of fiber and awesome vitamins. What's more, I find that if I have fresh fruit in the morning it seems to stop any sugar cravings from creeping in throughout the day.

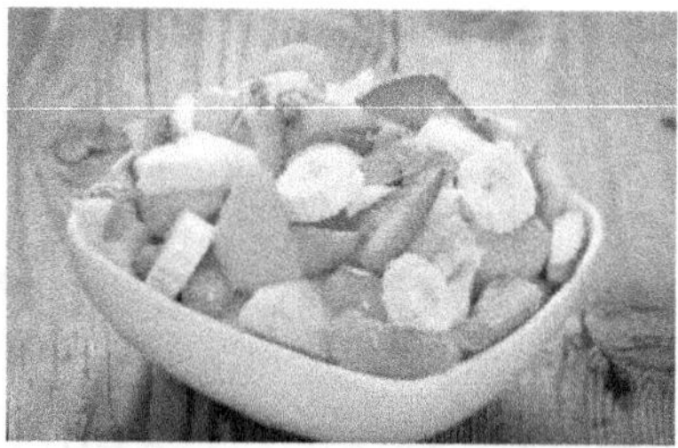

Serves: 3 (should be eaten within 3 days for maximum freshness)

Container: 3 sealable containers

Time: approximately 10 minutes

Nutritional info per serving:

- Calories: 176
- Fat: 0 grams
- Protein: 2 grams
- Carbs: 46 grams

Ingredients:

- 2 bananas, cut into chunks
- 4 large strawberries, cut into quarters
- 1 apple, core removed, flesh cut into small chunks
- 1 orange, cut into chunks
- 2 tbsp. honey
- 1 juicy lemon

Method:

1. Place the bananas, strawberries, apple, orange, honey, and juice of one lemon in a bowl and stir thoroughly to combine.
2. Divide the fruit salad between your 3 containers, cover, and store in the fridge.
3. For some extra protein, serve with plain Greek yogurt or a hard-boiled egg on the side.

BERRY, YOGURT, AND CHIA JARS

Chia seeds are full of fiber, protein, and fatty acids, which make them a filling and energy-giving breakfast ingredient. These jars are cooling, tangy, and slightly sweet thanks to the berry surprise at the bottom.

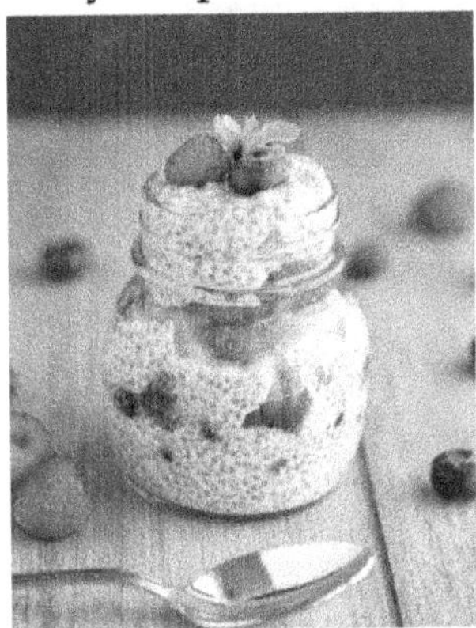

Serves: 5 jars (1 jar per serving)

Container: 5 glass jars with lids, or cups with cling wrap to cover

Time: approximately 10 minutes

Nutritional info per serving:

- Calories: 139
- Fat: 5 grams
- Protein: 4 grams
- Carbs: 17 grams

Ingredients:

- 2 cups mixed berries (frozen or fresh, I use frozen raspberries and blueberries)
- 6 tbsp. chia seeds
- 1 cup (8floz) almond milk
- ½ cup (4floz) cold water
- 1 tsp. cinnamon
- 1 tsp. vanilla extract
- 1 cup (8floz) plain, unsweetened yogurt

Method:

1. Divide the berries between your 5 jars or cups.
2. Place the chia seeds, almond milk, water, cinnamon, and vanilla extract into a small bowl and stir to combine.
3. Divide the chia seed mixture between the 5 jars, and spoon on top of the berries.
4. Divide the yogurt between the 5 jars and spoon on top of the chia mixture.

5. Sprinkle a little bit of cinnamon on top of the yogurt and place an extra berry on top (mostly for looks, but a pretty breakfast is an enjoyable one!).

6. Cover and place in the fridge.

SALMON AND EGG MUFFINS

A small amount of smoked salmon goes a long way. The fat content and rich saltiness is very satiating, while the eggs are filling without loading-up on carbs. These are great for when you just want a small breakfast.

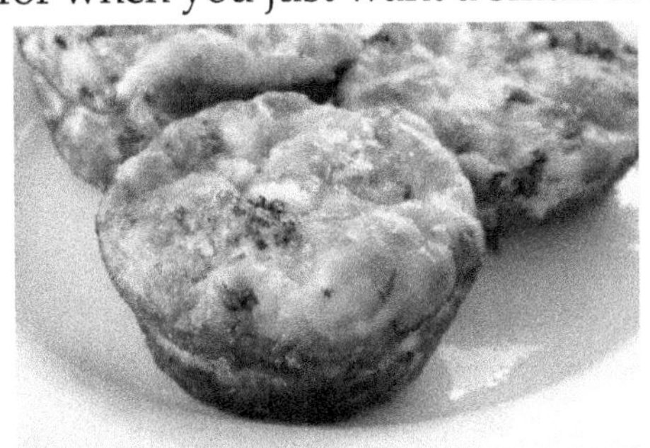

Serves: 6 muffins (1 muffin per serving)

Container: keep the muffins in an airtight container in the fridge

Time: approximately 15 minutes

Nutritional info per serving:

- Calories: 93
- Fat: 6 grams
- Protein: 8 grams
- Carbs: 1 gram

Ingredients:

- 4 eggs
- 1/3 cup milk
- Salt and pepper, to taste
- 1 ½ oz. smoked salmon, cut into small pieces
- 1 tbsp. finely chopped chives

Method:

1. Preheat the oven to 356 degrees Fahrenheit, and grease 6 muffin tin holes with some butter.
2. Place the eggs, milk, and a pinch of salt, and pepper into a small bowl and lightly beat to combine.
3. Divide the egg mixture between the 6 muffin holes, then divide the salmon between the muffins and place into each hole, gently pressing down to submerge in the egg mixture.
4. Sprinkle each muffin with chopped chives and place in the oven for about 8-10 minutes or until just set.
5. Leave to cool for about 5 minutes before turning out and storing in an airtight container in the fridge.

GREEN SMOOTHIE IN FREEZER PACKETS

Getting your greens in the morning always feels good, like you're checking something important off the list before you even leave the house! The blueberries might make this smoothie a little less green and more purple… but I still call it a green smoothie because of the spinach, kale, and green apples!

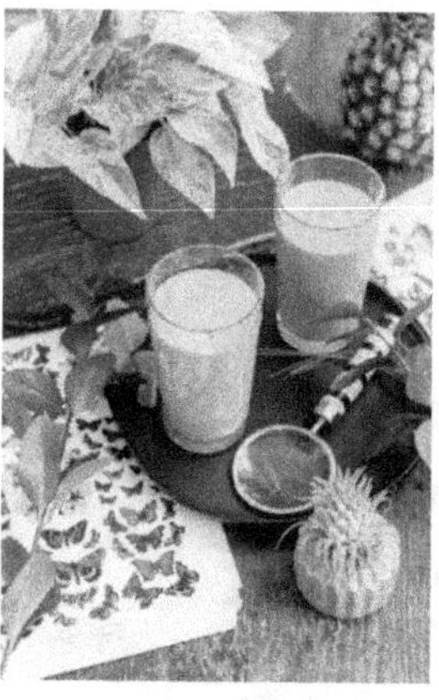

Serves: 7 freezer packets (one smoothie per packet)

Container: 7 small sealable, freezer-friendly bags

Time: approximately 10 minutes

Nutritional info per serving – with water added only:

- Calories: 105
- Fat: 3 grams
- Protein: 2 grams
- Carbs: 18 grams

Ingredients:

- 4 cups baby spinach leaves
- 2 cups chopped raw kale
- 1 avocado, flesh cut into chunks
- 2 green apples, skin on, cut into chunks
- 2 cups blueberries

Method:

1. Place the spinach, kale, avocado, apples, and blueberries into a bowl and stir to combine.
2. Divide the smoothie mixture between the 7 bags, seal, and place into the freezer.
3. To make the smoothie, empty the contents of one smoothie packet into the blender, and add enough water to suit your preferred smoothie consistency.

4. You may also use almond milk, coconut water, or yogurt, but keep in mind it will alter the nutritional value.

SOAKED OATS WITH VANILLA, DRIED FRUIT, AND NUTS

This is a recipe for very busy, active days, as the carb-count is generous and the energy rating is high! A great breakfast for after a morning run or gym session. Add some Greek yoghurt for extra protein, but remember it will change the nutritional index.

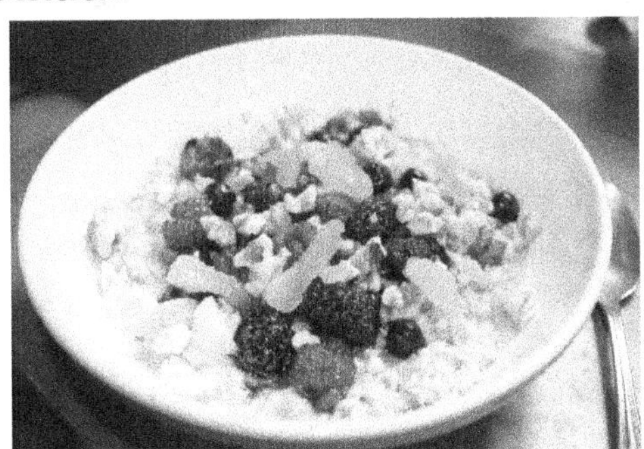

Serves: 4 soaked-oat jars

Container: 4 jars with lids, or 4 cups or ramekins with cling wrap to cover

Time: approximately 10 minutes

Nutritional info per serving:

- Calories: 300
- Fat: 11 grams
- Protein: 9 grams
- Carbs: 41 grams

Ingredients:

- 2 cups whole grain rolled oats
- 3 cups (24floz) almond milk
- 3 tsp. vanilla extract
- 4 prunes, chopped into small pieces
- 4 dates, chopped into small pieces
- 20 almonds, roughly chopped
- 12 walnuts, roughly chopped

Method:

1. Place the oats, almond milk, vanilla extract, prunes, dates, almonds, and walnuts into a bowl and stir to combine.
2. Divide the mixture between the 4 jars, seal or cover, then place in the fridge to soak overnight.

3. In the morning, if you find that the oats are a bit too stiff or dry for your liking, you can add a bit more almond milk to make them smoother.

TOASTED GRANOLA PACKS (TO TAKE TO WORK)

On those mornings when you have no time to eat breakfast at home, or you're not quite ready to eat yet, a portable pack of granola is the handiest option. Throw it in your bag and use the milk at your work (or take a little bottle of milk with you). And I'll admit, sometimes I like to snack on this granola dry, almost like a trail mix! Seeds provide healthy fats, and oats provide slow-release energy.

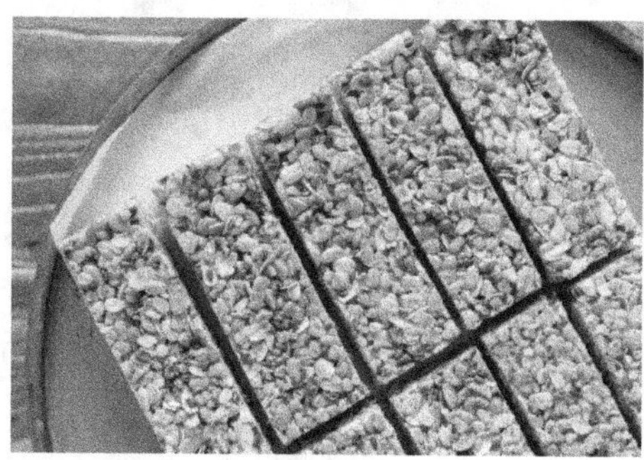

Serves: 7 packs (1 serving per pack)

Container: 7 small airtight containers or sealable bags

Time: approximately 15 minutes

Nutritional info per serving:

- Calories: 261
- Fat: 11 grams
- Protein: 12 grams
- Carbs: 33 grams

Ingredients:

- 2 tbsp. coconut oil
- 3 cups wholegrain rolled oats
- 4 tbsp. shredded coconut
- 3 tbsp. flaxseeds
- 3 tbsp. pumpkin seeds
- 3 tbsp. sunflower seeds
- 3 tbsp. chia seeds
- 10 dried apricots, chopped into small pieces
- 1 tsp. cinnamon
- ¼ tsp. sea salt

Method:

1. Heat the coconut oil in a large pan or pot over a medium heat.
2. Add the oats, coconut, flaxseeds, pumpkin seeds, sunflower seeds, chia seeds, dried apricots, cinnamon, and sea salt, stir to combine.
3. Keep stirring the mixture as it gently toasts for about 7 minutes or until golden and aromatic (it will smell like fresh baking!).
4. Leave in the pan to cool before filling your 7 bags or containers.
5. Store in the pantry.

DATE AND COCOA OATMEAL MIX

The reason for the inclusion of cocoa is pretty obvious…chocolate! Without the sugar and calories, of course. The dates provide a caramel-like sweetness to this amazing oatmeal breakfast, but if you're not a fan of dates, use any other dried fruit you like. The nutritional information provided here is only for the contents of the dry oatmeal mix, so you will have to add whichever milk you use to the calories and macros.

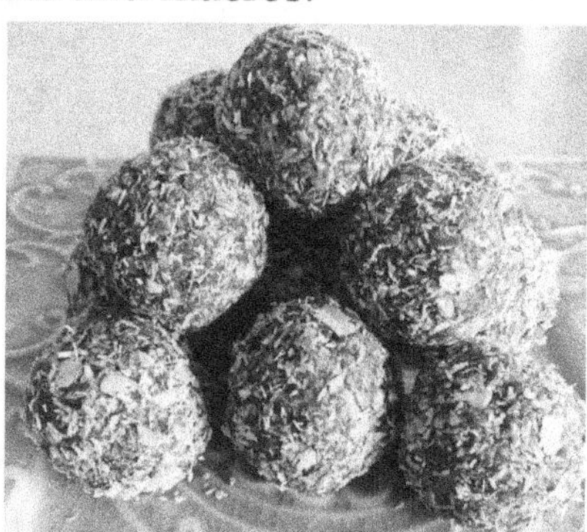

Serves: 7 servings of oatmeal

Container: you can either store this in one large container, or divide it into 7 single-serve containers

Time: approximately 10 minutes

Nutritional info per serving:

- Calories: 191
- Fat: 2 grams
- Protein: 7 grams
- Carbs: 37 grams

Ingredients:

- 4 cups wholegrain rolled oats
- 1 tbsp. unsweetened cocoa powder
- 15 dates, chopped into small pieces
- Pinch of salt

Method:

1. Place the oats, cocoa, dates, and salt into a bowl and stir to combine.
2. Place into one large container or 7 small containers and store in the pantry.
3. To make the oatmeal, place one serving of dry mix into a pot and add 1 and ¼ cups (10fl oz.) of water or milk, stir, and simmer until thick.

COCONUT AND ALMOND CHIA PUDDING

More chia seeds! I can't get enough of them. They're so filling and full of fiber (which is a major essential for weight loss). This recipe uses almond essence, chopped almonds, and coconut milk. It's a great recipe to choose when you feel like something a bit sweet and creamy.

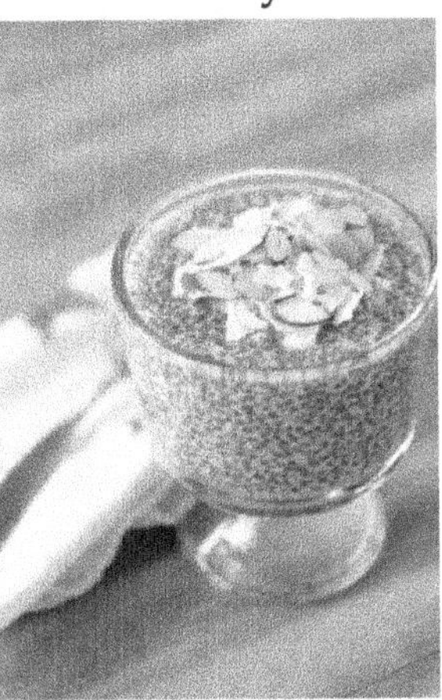

Serves: 4 puddings

Container: 4 jars or small bowls with a cling film to cover, or 4 containers with lids

Time: approximately 10 minutes (plus chilling overnight)

Nutritional info per serving:

- Calories: 296
- Fat: 19 grams
- Protein: 10 grams
- Carbs: 24 grams

Ingredients:

- 6 tbsp. chia seeds
- 1 cup wholegrain rolled oats
- 4 tbsp. desiccated coconut
- ½ tsp. almond essence
- ½ tsp. vanilla extract
- 4 cups (32fl oz.) unsweetened coconut milk
- 32 raw almonds, roughly chopped

Method:

1. Place the chia seeds, oats, desiccated coconut, almond essence, vanilla extract, coconut milk, and raw almonds into a bowl and stir to combine.
2. Divide between 4 jars or containers, cover, and place in the fridge overnight.

3. The chia seeds will expand and become gelatinous as they absorb moisture, so give the pudding a good stir before eating.

AVOCADO, KALE, AND MIXED BEAN BOWLS

Now a recipe for the lovers of savory breakfasts! Beans, avocado and kale are a super trio of fats, fiber, and good carbs. You can serve these bowls hot or cold, and they can even be eaten for lunch. If you need an extra dose of protein (perhaps after a session of heavy lifting) add a poached egg on top!

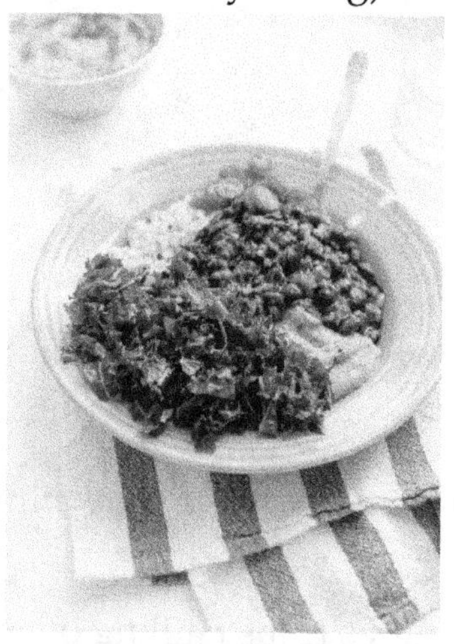

Serves: 4 bowls (1 serving per bowl)

Container: 4 airtight containers

Time: approximately 20 minutes

Nutritional info per serving:

- Calories: 290
- Fat: 11 grams
- Protein: 12 grams
- Carbs: 38 grams

Ingredients:

- ½ onion, finely chopped
- ½ tsp paprika
- 1 fresh tomato, chopped into chunks
- 1 can (14 oz.) black beans, drained
- 1 can (14 oz.) kidney beans, drained
- Salt and pepper, to taste
- 2 avocadoes, flesh sliced
- 2 cups chopped kale (chop it quite finely as kale tends to be tough)

Method:

1. Drizzle a small amount of olive oil into a pot and place over a low heat, add the onions, paprika, tomato, black beans, and kidney beans and stir to combine.
2. Simmer over medium heat for about 10 minutes until bubbling and thick, and add a pinch of salt and pepper to season.
3. Divide the bean mixture between 4 bowls and leave to cool slightly before placing the sliced avocado and kale on top.
4. Drizzle some extra olive oil over the top of the kale and avocado before covering with plastic wrap and placing into the fridge until needed.

NOT-SO-HUNGRY SNACK BAGS

You know those mornings when you just can't stomach a full-on breakfast, and you just want a little something to nibble on? That's what this recipe is for. No cooking involved here, just gathering a few simple dry ingredients and packing them into little bags or containers. Even though these snack bags are small, they provide a good dose of energy and healthy fat.

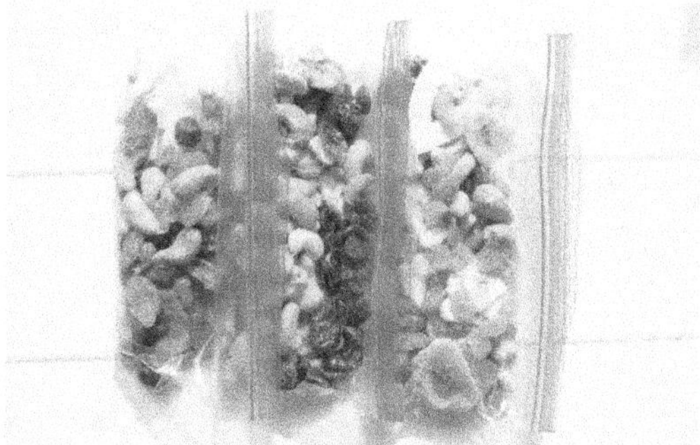

Serves: 7 snack bags (1 serving per snack bag)

Container: 7 sealable bags or airtight containers (small ones will do)

Time: approximately 10 minutes

Nutritional info per serving:

- Calories: 276
- Fat: 18 grams
- Protein: 10 grams
- Carbs: 24 grams

Ingredients:

- 14 prunes
- 14 dried apricots
- 14 whole walnuts
- ½ cup raw almonds
- 14 macadamia nuts
- ¼ cup pumpkin seeds

Method:

1. Divide each ingredient into 7 containers or bags, seal, and place in the pantry. Very easy!
2. If you like, you could make the pieces smaller by chopping the dates, prunes, and nuts into small pieces, almost like trail mix.
3. Keep these bags in your handbag or office desk for a healthy snack when the cravings hit.

Fresh, cold, creamy Greek yogurt is one of my favorite things to eat for breakfast, especially when I know I need some extra probiotics and some protein to help my muscles repair from a lifting session. While the pre-flavored yoghurt varieties are often full of refined sugar, this version is flavored by you, at home, with ingredients you can trust. Mangoes, honey, and lime…you could even eat it as a dessert treat!

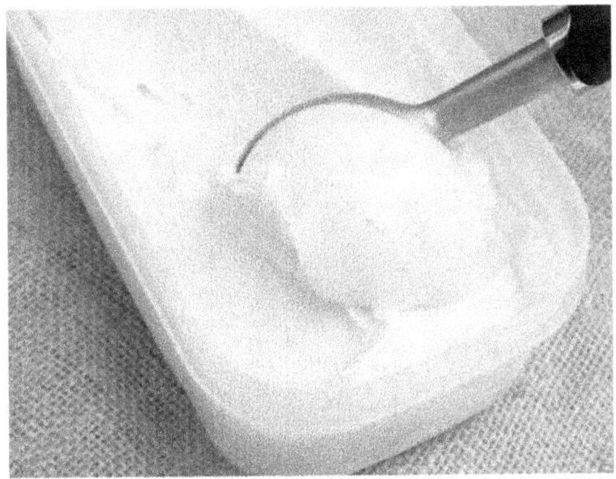

Serves: 5 servings

Container: 5 small airtight containers

Time: approximately 10 minutes

Nutritional info per serving:

- Calories: 266
- Fat: 14 grams
- Protein: 7 grams
- Carbs: 30 grams

Ingredients:

- 2 mangoes, flesh removed and cut into small pieces
- 3 cups (24fl oz.) unsweetened Greek yogurt
- 1 tbsp. honey
- 1 lime

Method:

1. Place half of the mango into a blender, or use a stick blender, and blend to puree.
2. Place the blended mango, remaining mango chunks, yogurt, honey, and grated zest of one lime into a bowl and stir to combine.
3. Divide between 5 containers, cover, and store in the fridge.
4. For an extra treat, sprinkle a few chopped almonds or some desiccated coconut on top before eating.

PRE-MADE BANANA PANCAKES

These pancakes do not contain any sugar, flour or butter! Bananas, eggs and ground almonds are the main ingredients. Bananas provide potassium and sweetness; eggs add the protein, and ground almonds contain healthy fats. Fry them up during your prep session, store them in the fridge, and then zap them in the microwave or frying pan to heat before serving.

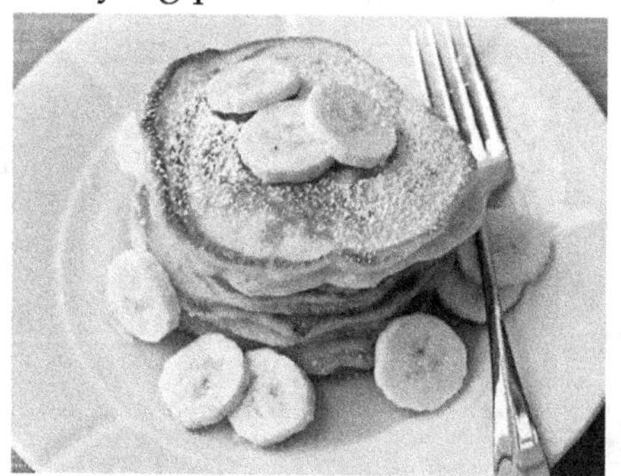

Serves: 15 pancakes (5 servings, 3 pancakes per serving)

Container: 1 airtight container to store all of the pancakes is ideal

Time: approximately 25 minutes

Nutritional info per serving:

- Calories: 170
- Fat: 11 grams
- Protein: 6 grams
- Carbs: 14 grams

Ingredients:

- 2 large bananas, peeled and cut into chunks
- 3 eggs
- ½ cup ground almonds
- 1 tsp. vanilla extract
- ½ tsp baking powder
- Coconut oil, for frying

Method:

1. Place the bananas, eggs, ground almonds, vanilla extract, and baking powder into a bowl and mash using a fork, handheld stick blender, or potato masher until smooth and combined.
2. Drizzle some coconut oil in a non-stick frying pan and place over a medium heat until the oil gets hot.
3. Place a scoop of pancake mixture into the hot pan and cook on both sides until golden and cooked through.

4. Place the cooked pancakes in your airtight container and store in the fridge.

5. Before eating the next morning, simply heat the pancakes in the microwave or in a dry, hot frying pan until heated through.

6. Serve with yogurt and fruit, or simply eat plain!

SPINACH, MUSHROOM AND FETA BREAKFAST PIES

These pies are SO light in calories, you can have them as a snack on the side of a more robust breakfast. They are a great way to get extra protein and a dose of greens in the morning. The feta cheese adds creaminess and a tart saltiness to satisfy your taste buds.

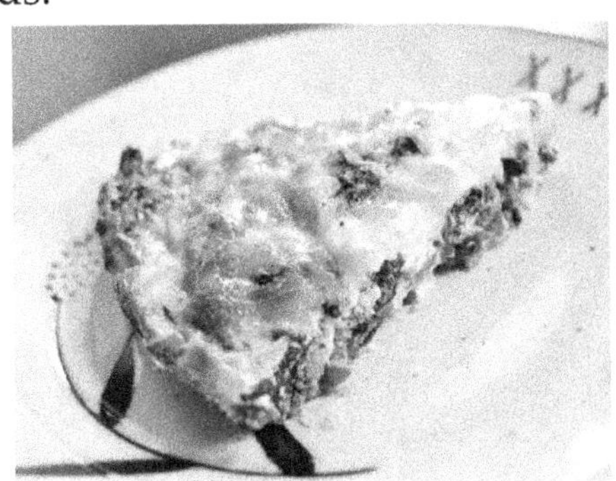

Serves: 1 large pie to be cut into 8 pieces (8 servings)

Container: store in the fridge in a large airtight container with baking paper to separate the layers of pie slices so they don't stick together

Time: approximately 25 minutes

Nutritional info per serving:

- Calories: 67
- Fat: 5 grams
- Protein: 5 grams
- Carbs: 1 gram

Ingredients:

- 5 eggs
- 2 cups chopped spinach
- 1 cup sliced mushrooms (any kind)
- 2 oz. feta cheese, cut into small pieces, or crumbled
- Salt and pepper, to taste

Method:

1. Preheat the oven to 356 degrees Fahrenheit, and grease a rectangular pie or casserole dish with cooking spray or butter.

2. Place the eggs, spinach, mushrooms, feta, salt, and pepper into a
    bowl and whisk to combine.
3. Pour the mixture into the greased dish and place into the oven to
    bake for about 10 minutes until just set.
4. Leave to cool before slicing into 8 pieces and placing into an
    airtight container.
5. Store in the fridge.

BELL PEPPER AND BEAN BURRITOS

These burritos are ideal for those power days when you've got lots of exercise, work, and running around to do. They are packed with fiber and protein from the beans and eggs, and the sweetness of softened bell peppers. Fresh cilantro and red chili offer a hit of fresh flavor and bright color.

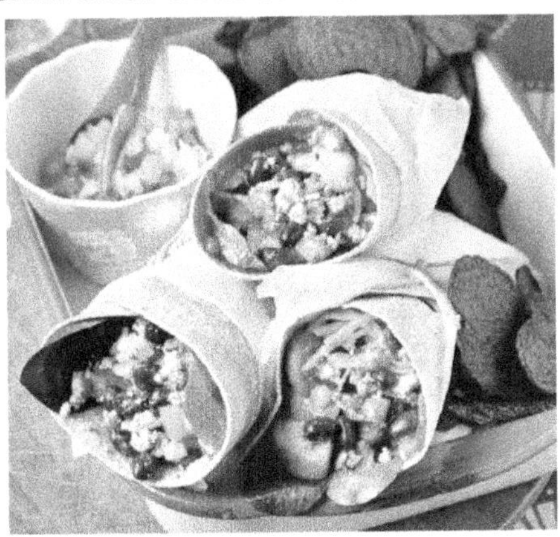

Serves: 4 burritos (1 burrito is 1 serving)

Container: 4 single-serve airtight containers, or 1 large one to store all 4 burritos

Time: approximately 20 minutes

Nutritional info per serving:

- Calories: 310
- Fat: 8 grams
- Protein: 14 grams
- Carbs: 45 grams

Ingredients:

- 2 garlic cloves, finely chopped
- 2 red bell peppers, finely sliced
- 1 tsp. paprika
- ½ tsp. chili powder
- 1 can (14 oz.) black beans, drained
- Salt and pepper, to taste
- 2 eggs, lightly beaten
- 4 small flour or corn tortillas
- Fresh cilantro, chopped
- ½ fresh red chili, finely chopped

Method:

1. Drizzle some olive oil into a frying pan and heat it over a medium heat.

2. Add the garlic, bell peppers, paprika, and chili powder, sauté until the bell peppers are soft.
3. Add the black beans and a pinch of salt and pepper, stir to combine, continue to sauté.
4. Move the bean and bell pepper mixture to one side of the pan and pour the lightly-beaten eggs on the other side, stir them as they scramble until just cooked.
5. Turn off the heat and lay your tortillas on a board.
6. Fill each tortilla with bell pepper, beans, and eggs.
7. Sprinkle with cilantro and fresh chili, and tightly wrap them.
8. Carefully place the burritos into your container/s, cover, and store in the fridge.

CHORIZO AND SWEET POTATO HASH

Okay, you got me… chorizo isn't a "weight loss" food, but it's tasty, salty, and full of flavor to satisfy you throughout the morning. A little bit of chorizo sausage is not going to sabotage your weight-loss goals, so go ahead and enjoy it! Sweet potato provides fiber and good carbs, and eggs offer that ever-important protein. Slice this hash into 4 pieces, store them away in the fridge, and eat hot or cold for a tasty, savory breakfast.

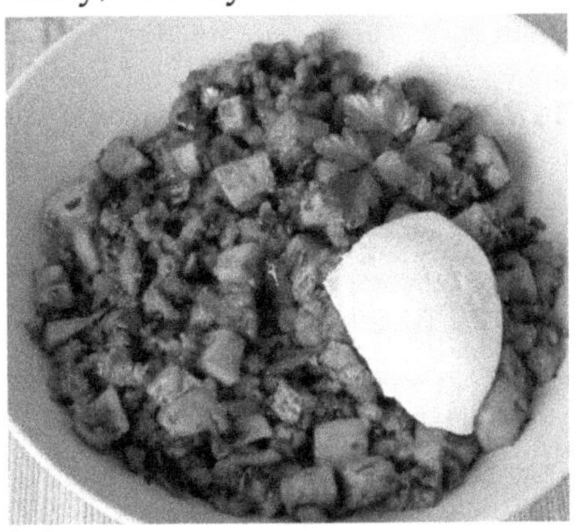

Serves: 4

Container: 1 large airtight container to store all 4 pieces, or 4 single-serve containers

Time: approximately 25 minutes

Nutritional info per serving:

- Calories: 236
- Fat: 11 grams
- Protein: 12 grams
- Carbs: 24 grams

Ingredients:

- 3 cups sweet potato, cubed (about 2 large sweet potatoes)
- 1 chorizo sausage, sliced
- 1 cup spinach leaves, chopped
- 3 eggs, lightly beaten

Method:

1. Place the sweet potatoes into a pot and cover it with water, boil over a medium heat and leave to simmer, uncovered, until the sweet potatoes are soft but not mushy.
2. Drizzle some olive oil into a non-stick frying pan and heat it over medium heat.
3. Add the chorizo to the hot frying pan and sauté for a few minutes until crispy and the oil has melted out.

4. Place the sweet potatoes into the frying pan and stir them as they are sautéing for a few minutes; it's okay if you crush them a bit.

5. Add the spinach to the pan and stir into the sweet potatoes and chorizo until wilted.

6. Pour the eggs over the top of the sweet potato mixture and allow them to seep through the potatoes, make little holes with a wooden spoon to let the eggs combine with the other ingredients if you need to.

7. Cook the hash for a few minutes or until the eggs have just set.

8. Cut into 4 pieces and either store in one large container, or in 4 single-serve containers.

9. Place into the fridge to store until needed.

10. Eat hot or cold!

BLUEBERRY AND MINT PARFAITS

Blueberries are full of antioxidants and healthy carbs. Not only they are nutritious, but also tasty and pretty (for some reason I love to eat foods that look pretty on the plate, it makes them taste yummier somehow!). Mint is invigorating and refreshing, providing a burst of color. Of course, I have to add oats to the yoghurt-base of this parfait, they are too filling and wholesome to leave out.

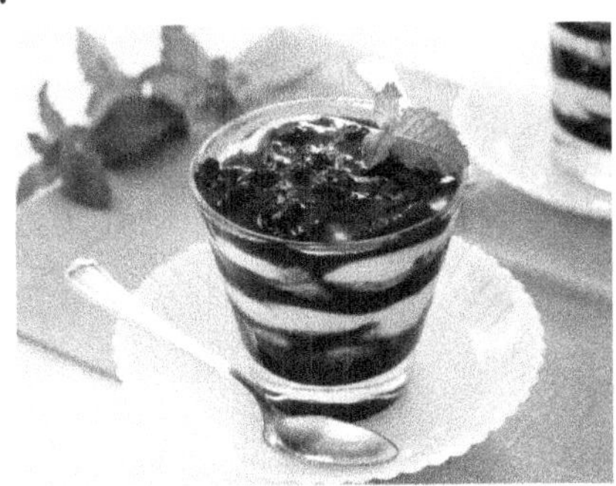

Serves: 4 parfaits

Container: 4 glass bowls, ramekins, cups or airtight containers if transporting the parfait to work

Time: approximately 10 minutes

Nutritional info per serving:

- Calories: 272
- Fat: 8 grams
- Protein: 10 grams
- Carbs: 25 grams

Ingredients:

- 1 ½ cups wholegrain rolled oats
- 1 cup (8fl oz.) almond milk
- 2 cups (16fl oz.) unsweetened Greek yogurt
- 1 cup fresh blueberries (can also use frozen, no need to thaw first)
- 4 small fresh mint leaves, finely chopped

Method:

1. Place the oats and almond milk into a bowl and stir together to combine (this helps the oats to soften).
2. Spoon the oat and almond milk mixture evenly into your 4 containers.
3. Place a drop of yogurt into each container on top of the oats (use half of the yogurt as you'll be adding another layer of it).
4. Divide half of the blueberries between the 4 containers and sprinkle on top of the yogurt.

5. Add another layer of yogurt and then another layer of blueberries (you can use them all up at this stage).
6. Sprinkle the fresh mint on top of each parfait.
7. Cover and place in the fridge to store until needed!

PEANUT BUTTER AND BANANA BREAKFAST CAKE

Do not panic, this is not a "cake" in the sense we usually think of cakes! As much as I would love to offer a regular cake for breakfast, it doesn't really help the weight loss cause. This "cake" is made of bananas, peanut butter, eggs, almond flour and almond milk – healthy and nutritious ingredients, full of energy, fat, and protein. You can freeze slices of this cake and pull them out when you're in a pinch.

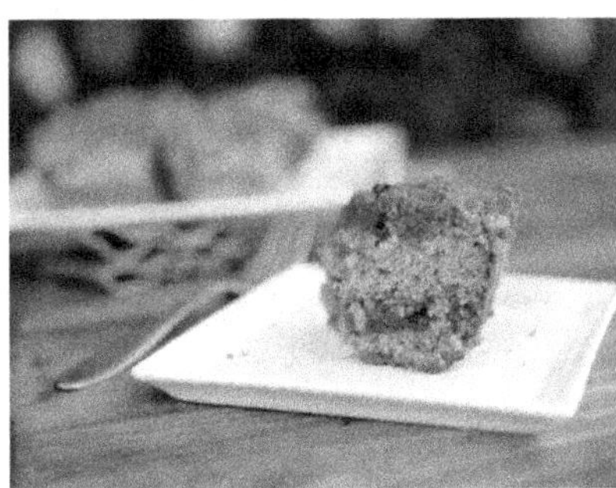

Serves: 8 slices (1 serving per slice)

Container: 1 large container or 8 single-serve containers if taking to work

Time: approximately 20 minutes

Nutritional info per serving:

- Calories: 200
- Fat: 12 grams
- Protein: 7 grams
- Carbs: 16 grams

Ingredients:

- 3 bananas, mashed
- 4 tbsp. natural peanut butter (crunchy or smooth, either one is fine)
- 3 eggs
- 1 cup almond flour (this can be expensive so simply use whole-meal gluten-free flour if you like)
- 1 cup (8fl oz.) almond milk
- 1 tsp. baking powder
- 1 tsp. vanilla extract

Method:

1. Preheat the oven to 350 degrees Fahrenheit and prepare a baking dish by lining with some baking paper.
2. Place the bananas, peanut butter, eggs, almond flour, almond milk, baking powder, and vanilla extract into a bowl and stir to combine.
3. Pour the mixture into the prepared baking dish and introduce into the oven, bake for approximately 15 minutes or until just set.

4. Leave to cool before slicing into 8 pieces and storing in an airtight container in the fridge.

5. Eat hot or cold!

SPINACH AND ZUCCHINI BREAKFAST PIE WITH OPTIONAL SMOKED FISH

In a perfect world, greens should be consumed at every meal – they are the best source of essential micronutrients to keep you glowing and healthy. I have added "optional" smoked fish to this recipe because I understand that not everyone can feel like eating fish at breakfast time! Personally? I adore smoked trout so I always add it to this breakfast pie. Note: the nutritional information includes the smoked fish.

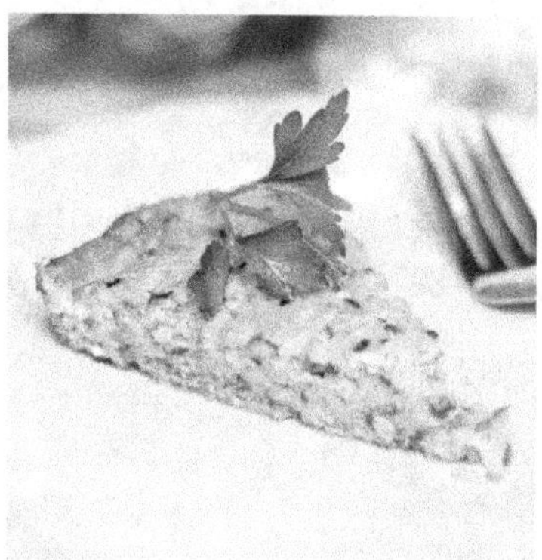

Serves: 8 slices (1 serving per slice)

Container: 1 large container or 8 single-serve containers if transporting to work

Time: approximately 25 minutes

Nutritional info per serving:

- Calories: 150
- Fat: 4 grams
- Protein: 11 grams
- Carbs: 10 grams

Ingredients:

- 3 cups baby spinach leaves, roughly chopped
- 2 large zucchinis, sliced
- 5 eggs, lightly beaten
- ½ cup (4floz) milk
- ½ cup whole-meal flour
- ½ tsp baking powder
- 7 oz. smoked fish, flaked (optional)
- Salt and pepper, to taste

Method:

1. Preheat the oven to 356 degrees Fahrenheit, and prepare a baking tray by lining it with some baking paper.
2. Drizzle some olive oil into a frying pan and heat it over medium heat.
3. Add the spinach and zucchini and sauté until wilted and softened.
4. In a bowl, whisk together the eggs, milk, flour, and baking powder until smooth.
5. Add the cooked spinach, zucchini, and flaked smoke fish (if using) into the bowl and stir to combine, then add a pinch of salt and pepper to season.
6. Pour into the prepared tray and introduce into the oven for approximately 15 minutes or until just set.
7. Leave to cool then cut into 8 pieces and store in the fridge!
8. Eat hot or cold.

STRAWBERRY, PUMPKIN SEED AND COCONUT OAT BAKED CRISP

This is another "cake"-inspired breakfast, but without the empty calories. Full of good fats and healthy fiber, this is a naturally sweet and tasty breakfast for eating on the go, or in a bowl with some Greek yoghurt for more protein.

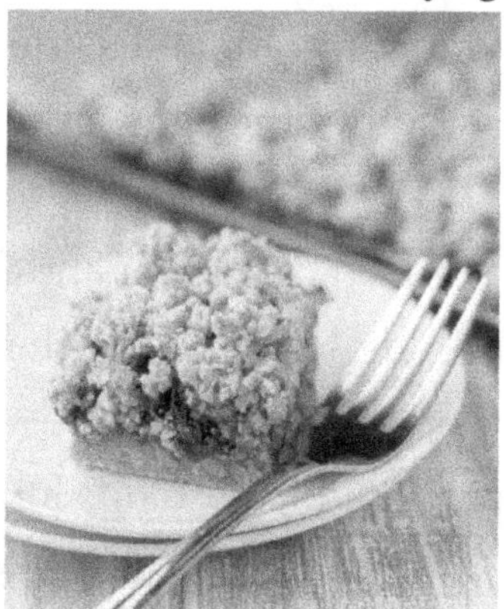

Serves: 8 slices (1 serving per slice)

Container: 1 large container or 8 single-serve containers if transporting to work

Time: approximately 25 minutes

Nutritional info per serving:

- Calories: 160
- Fat: 7 grams
- Protein: 7 grams
- Carbs: 19 grams

Ingredients:

- 3 tbsp. pumpkin seeds
- 2 cups wholegrain rolled oats
- ½ cup desiccated coconut
- 1 tsp. cinnamon
- 1 egg, lightly beaten
- 2 tbsp. honey
- ½ cup (4loz) almond milk
- ½ tsp. baking powder
- 1 cup fresh strawberries, cut into quarters

Method:

1. Preheat the oven to 356 degrees Fahrenheit, and prepare a baking try by lining it with baking paper.

2. Place the pumpkin seeds, oats, coconut, cinnamon, egg, honey, almond milk, and baking powder into a bowl and stir to combine; it will be thick – that's okay!

3. Press half of the mixture into the lined tray and then place the strawberries on the top in an even layer, press the rest of the oat mixture over the strawberries.

4. Place the tray into the oven and bake for approximately 15-20 minutes or until golden.

5. Leave to cool before slicing into 8 pieces and storing in the fridge or freezer until needed!

BREAKFAST TACOS WITH EGGS, BELL PEPPER AND MUSHROOMS

I like to think of these breakfast tacos as something to make when I know I will have guests to cater to, who might like something a little more exciting than a regular breakfast. They are tasty and joyful, but still conform to the healthy-eating guidelines I have set for myself and my weight-loss goals. For low-carb days, just leave out the tortilla and have the eggs and veggies!

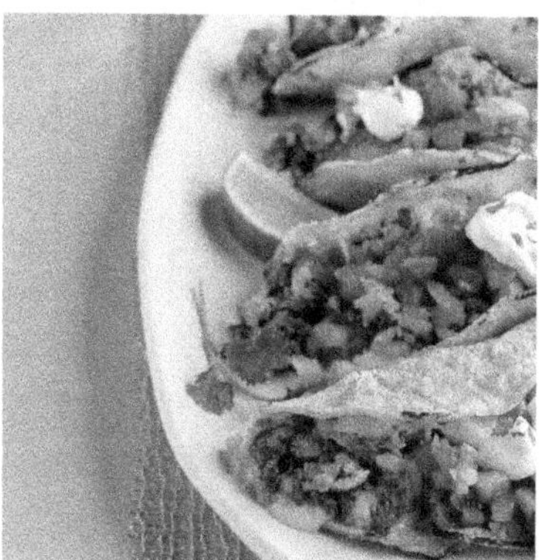

Serves: 8 tacos (2 tacos per serving, so 4 servings)

Container: you can store all 8 in one large container or use 4 smaller containers to store 2

Time: approximately 20 minutes

Nutritional info per serving:

- Calories: 387
- Fat: 15 grams
- Protein: 22 grams
- Carbs: 47 grams

Ingredients:

- 2 red bell peppers, core and seeds removed, flesh sliced
- 4 large Portobello mushrooms, sliced
- Salt and pepper, to taste
- 6 eggs, lightly beaten
- 8 whole-meal tortilla wraps
- 4 tbsp. plain Greek yogurt
- 1 fresh red chili, finely chopped
- Handful of fresh cilantro, roughly chopped

Method:

1. Drizzle some olive oil into a pan and heat it over a medium heat.
2. Add the bell peppers, mushrooms, and a pinch of salt and pepper, sauté until soft.

3. Move the veggies to one side of the pan and pour the eggs on the other side, stirring them with a wooden spoon continuously as they scramble, cook until just set.
4. Take the pan off the heat and place your tortillas on a large cutting board.
5. Spread a small amount of Greek yogurt along each wrap, then divide the bell peppers and mushrooms between each wrap, placing them on top of the yogurt, then do the same with the eggs.
6. Finish with a sprinkle of chili and cilantro on top of each one!
7. Carefully fold them up and place them in your containers.
8. Store in the fridge until needed!
9. These are best eaten cold due to the added Greek yogurt.

SALMON, KALE, RICOTTA AND EGG FRY-PAN CAKE

Smoked salmon and ricotta are rich and full of good fats, so they can be eaten in small quantities in order to reap the benefits. Kale is, of course, full of minerals and fiber, and eggs are our protein savior.

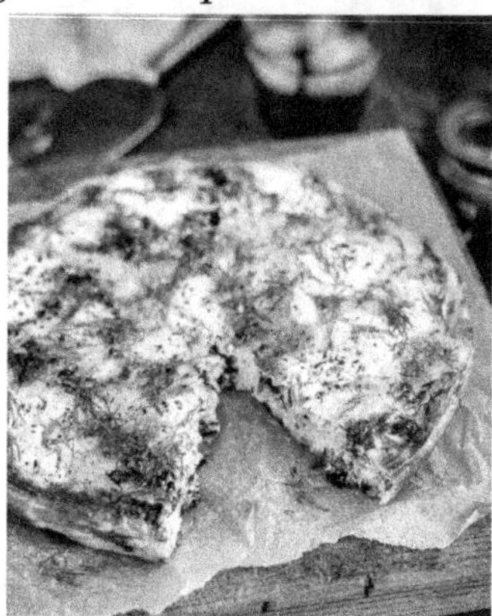

Serves: 6 slices

Container: you can store all 6 slices in one container and take them out as you need them, or use 6 small containers if you are transporting the slices to work

Time: approximately 15 minutes

Nutritional info per serving:

- Calories: 120
- Fat: 7 grams
- Protein: 11 grams
- Carbs: 2 grams

Ingredients:

- 5 eggs, lightly beaten
- 4 oz. ricotta cheese
- 2 cups kale, finely sliced
- Salt and pepper, to taste
- 2 oz. smoked salmon, cut into small pieces

Method:

1. Place the eggs, ricotta, kale, salt, and pepper into a bowl and whisk to combine.
2. Drizzle some olive oil into a non-stick fry pan and heat it over a medium heat.
3. Pour the egg mixture in the frying pan and sprinkle the smoked salmon pieces over the top.
4. Cook for approximately 7 minutes or until just set.
5. Leave to cool before slicing into 6 pieces and storing in the fridge until needed!

HEALTHY BREAKFAST CRUMBLE WITH STONE FRUIT AND BERRIES

Yes, this is absolutely a fruit crumble – BUT, it doesn't have the flour, butter and sugar of a dessert crumble. And it is a perfect choice for when the stone fruits are in season! I use peaches and nectarines, but you could also use plums and any other yummy stone fruits you like. Be creative with the berries too, use a mixture!

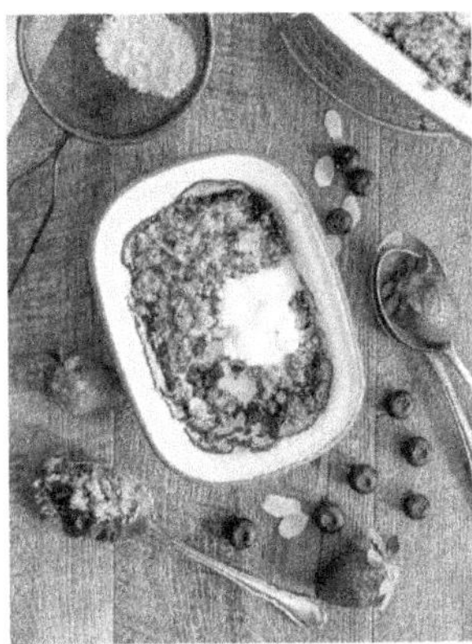

Serves: 8 (small servings)

Container: I like to store the entire thing in a large airtight container and just take slices out when I need them, but you could divide them up and store in 8 small containers if you wish.

Time: approximately 35 minutes

Nutritional info per serving:

- Calories: 213
- Fat: 10 grams
- Protein: 5 grams
- Carbs: 31 grams

Ingredients:

- 3 ripe peaches, stones removed, flesh cut into slices
- 4 ripe nectarines, stones removed, flesh cut into slices
- 2 cups frozen mixed berries
- 1 ½ cups wholegrain rolled oats
- 1/3 cup sliced almonds
- 1 tbsp. chia seeds
- 1 tsp. cinnamon
- 1/3 cup desiccated coconut
- 2 tbsp. coconut oil
- 2 tbsp. honey

Method:

1. Preheat the oven to 356 degrees Fahrenheit.
2. Place the sliced peaches, nectarines, and berries into a large rectangular baking dish and stir to combine.
3. Add the oats, almonds, chia seeds, cinnamon, desiccated coconut, coconut oil, and honey into a bowl and stir to combine.
4. Sprinkle the crumble over the fruits and introduce into the oven to bake for approximately 30 minutes or until the crumble is golden and the fruits are soft.
5. Leave to cool before slicing into 8 slices and store in the fridge until needed.

LUNCH

These lunch recipes could also be used as dinner recipes, as they contain plenty of veggies and lean proteins. Grains such as quinoa and brown rice are also featured in this section, as it's important to eat slow-releasing energy sources at lunchtime to keep you alert and full throughout the afternoon. If you are exercising a lot as part of your weight-loss attempts, then please don't forget to eat enough throughout the day! That means a wholesome lunch. You can go easy on the carbs at dinnertime if you wish, but don't be shy to chow down on plenty of nutrients for your midday meal.

QUINOA AND FRESH GREENS SALAD

Many people assume that quinoa is a specialty ingredient, but it's so common these days it's just like rice or bread! It can be slightly pricey, but you don't need to use much. This salad is very simple: quinoa, lettuce, spinach, and green bell peppers, with a wee bit of feta to make it special.

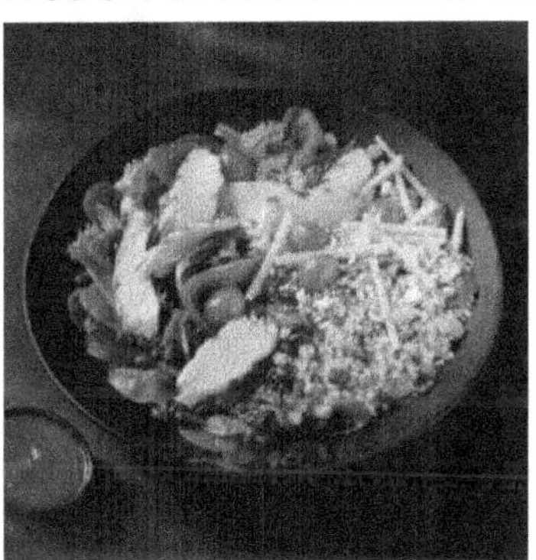

Serves: 4

Container: you will need 4 airtight containers or lunchboxes

Time: approximately 25 minutes

Nutritional info per serving:

- Calories: 450
- Fat: 9 grams
- Protein: 17 grams
- Carbs: 65 grams

Ingredients:

- 1 cup dry quinoa
- 1 ½ cups (12floz) salt-reduced chicken broth/stock
- 3 cups shredded lettuce (use any, I use iceberg)
- 2 cups baby spinach leaves
- 2 green bell peppers, core and seeds removed, sliced
- 3 oz. feta cheese, cut into small chunks

- Salt and pepper, to taste

Method:

1. Thoroughly rinse the quinoa in a sieve to remove the bitter outer layer.
2. Bring the chicken broth to a boil in a small pot and add the quinoa, stir to combine then turn the heat down to a simmer, cover, and cook for 12-15 minutes or until the liquid has evaporated and the quinoa is soft.
3. Divide the cooked quinoa between your 4 containers, then divide the lettuce, spinach, bell peppers and feta between the containers and stir to combine.
4. Sprinkle with salt and pepper and drizzle with olive oil to finish.
5. Cover and place into the fridge until needed!

ROASTED VEGGIE SALAD

Easy, classic, tasty and filling. A roasted veggie salad is what I would turn to when all I want to do is throw a tray in the oven and be done with it! Added seeds provide extra fats and energy.

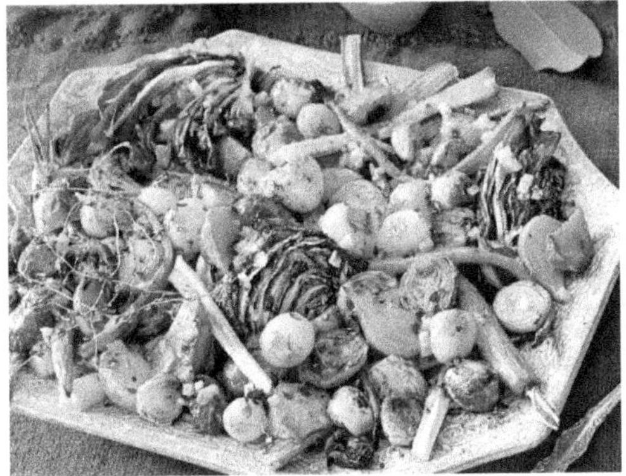

Serves: 4

Container: you will need 4 airtight containers

Time: approximately 30 minutes

Nutritional info per serving:

- Calories: 300
- Fat: 16 grams
- Protein: 9 grams
- Carbs: 31 grams

Ingredients:

- 2 cups cubed butternut squash (I keep the skin on but you can remove it if you wish)
- 2 cups cubed sweet potato
- 2 carrots, chopped into chunks
- 2 large Portobello mushrooms, thickly sliced
- 2 large zucchinis, cut into chunks
- 1 head of broccoli, cut into florets
- 2 tbsp. sunflower seeds
- 2 tbsp. pumpkin seeds
- 3 tbsp. olive oil (I've added the oil in here because it's quite a lot and it adjusts the calorie count)
- Salt and pepper, to taste

Method:

1. Preheat the oven to 356 degrees Fahrenheit, and prepare a tray by lining it with baking paper.

2. Place all vegetables and seeds on the tray and add a sprinkle of salt
   and pepper.
3. Combine the ingredients together with your hands, making sure
   everything gets coated in olive oil.
4. Place into the oven and bake for approximately 30 minutes or until
   the veggies are soft and the seeds are toasted.
5. Divide between 4 containers, cover and place into the fridge until
   needed.

GRILLED CHICKEN WITH SWEET POTATOES AND ASPARAGUS

Lean protein and healthy carbs is a lunch of champions. It's simple, yes, but it is delicious. High-energy days with weight training call for a lunch just like this one. You only need an oven and one tray to complete this dish!

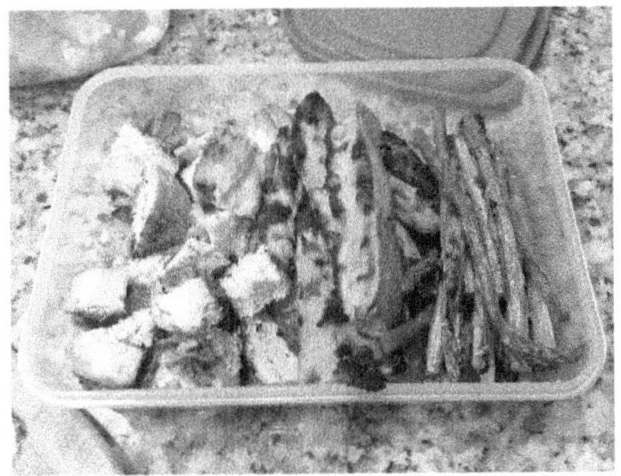

Serves: 4

Container: you will need 4 airtight containers

Time: approximately 35 minutes

Nutritional info per serving:

- Calories: 280
- Fat: 13 grams
- Protein: 28 grams
- Carbs: 11 grams

Ingredients:

- 4 small chicken breasts
- 1 large sweet potato, cut into chunks
- 16 spears of asparagus, tough ends removed
- 2 tbsp. olive oil
- 1 tsp. dried rosemary
- Salt and pepper, to taste

Method:

1. Preheat the oven to 356 degrees Fahrenheit, and prepare a tray by lining it with baking paper.
2. Place the chicken, sweet potato, asparagus, olive oil, rosemary, salt, and pepper on the tray and combine with your hands until everything is coated in oil and seasoning.
3. Introduce into the oven and bake for approximately 30 minutes or until the chicken is cooked through and the sweet potatoes are soft.
4. Divide between 4 containers, cover, and place into the fridge until needed.

5. Eat hot or cold!

BROWN RICE AND TUNA BOWLS

Brown rice and canned tuna – a student's dream! Affordable and nutritious, this is a lunch for tight budgets and energetic days. Best eaten cold for a Summery and refreshing lunchtime munch.

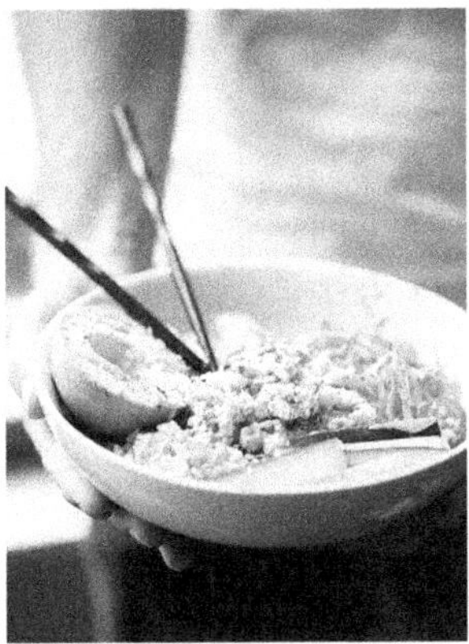

Serves: 4

Container: you will need 4 airtight containers

Time: approximately 25 minutes

Nutritional info per serving:

- Calories: 450
- Fat: 5 grams
- Protein: 23 grams
- Carbs: 78 grams

Ingredients:

- 2 cups dry brown rice
- 4 small cans of unflavored tuna (the single-serve cans)
- 1 carrot, peeled and chopped into small pieces
- 1 red bell pepper, core and seeds removed, cut into small pieces
- 1 cup chopped cucumber
- 1 tbsp. balsamic vinegar

Method:

1. Add the brown rice to a pot and pour 3 ½ cups of water and a pinch of salt, bring to a boil and then reduce the heat to a simmer, leave covered until the water has evaporated and the rice is soft (but still with a bite!).
2. Divide the cooked rice between 4 containers and add the contents of one tuna can into each, divide the carrot, bell pepper, cucumber and balsamic vinegar between the 4 containers and stir to combine with the rice.
3. Cover and place into the fridge to store until needed!

PITA POCKETS WITH LAMB AND SALAD

Whole-meal pita pockets with lamb and salad greens, with a drizzle of plain yoghurt - this is the kind of lunch you'll want to eat as soon as you get to work! But you'll just have to wait.

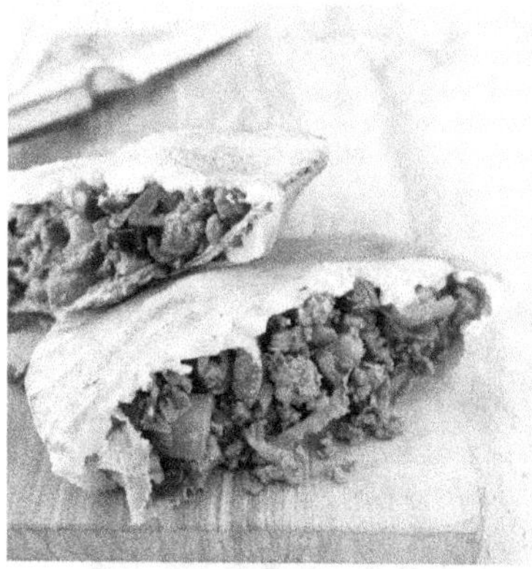

Serves: 4

Container: you will need 4 airtight containers

Time: approximately 20 minutes

Nutritional info per serving:

- Calories: 520
- Fat: 27 grams
- Protein: 37 grams
- Carbs: 32 grams

Ingredients:

- 12 oz. lamb steaks, cut into cubes
- 1 tsp. ground cumin
- Salt and pepper, to taste
- 4 whole-meal pita breads
- 2 cups salad greens (mixed kale, lettuce and arugula is ideal)
- 4 tbsp. plain yogurt
- 1 lemon, cut into quarters

Method:

1. Pour some olive oil in a frying pan and heat it over medium heat.
2. Add the lamb, cumin, salt and pepper and stir to combine, sauté for about 7 minutes or until the lamb cubes are cooked but still a little pink.
3. Make a slit in each pita bread and fill each one with mixed salad greens, lamb, and a drizzle of yogurt.

4. Transfer the filled pitas to 4 containers and place a lemon quarter in each one so you can squeeze it over the pita when you're ready to eat!

5. Cover the containers and store in the fridge until needed.

STICKY CHICKEN AND BROCCOLI PREP BOWLS

Chicken and broccoli – the dieter's staple! But this dish is far from bland or boring. Soy sauce and honey make a sticky sauce for the chicken, and sesame oil jazzes-up the broccoli for a tasty and filling lunch suitable for any day of the week.

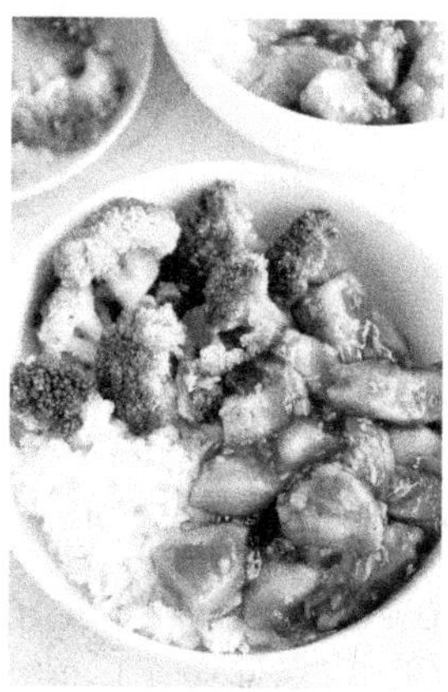

Serves: 4

Container: you will need 4 airtight containers

Time: approximately 30 minutes

Nutritional info per serving:

- Calories: 298
- Fat: 12 grams
- Protein: 31 grams
- Carbs: 19 grams

Ingredients:

- 2 tbsp. honey
- 2 tsp. soy sauce (tamari is best)
- 4 boneless, skinless chicken thighs
- 1 head of broccoli, cut into florets
- 1 tsp. sesame oil

Method:

1. Pour some olive oil in a frying pan and heat it over medium heat.
2. Add the honey and soy sauce, place the chicken thighs into the pan and stir to coat in soy and honey, sauté for approximately 15 minutes or until the chicken is almost cooked.
3. Add the broccoli to the pan, increase the heat to high, splash a few teaspoons of water into the pan and immediately place cover with a lid – this will steam the broccoli.

4. Once the water has evaporated, remove the lid and make sure that the chicken has cooked through and the broccoli is cooked yet crunchy.
5. Drizzle the sesame oil over the broccoli before dividing the chicken and broccoli between 4 containers.
6. Cover and store in the fridge until needed!

I just had to add a recipe in here which was just a teeny and tiny bit naughty. After all, a cheat meal here and this is not going to ruin your weight loss! This recipe is still tasty and uses whole, real ingredients, but it's quite bread and cheese-rich, so it's definitely one to keep up your sleeve until you're really craving for some comfort food. Prepare the sandwiches the night/s before, then throw them on the grill or in the sandwich press before eating.

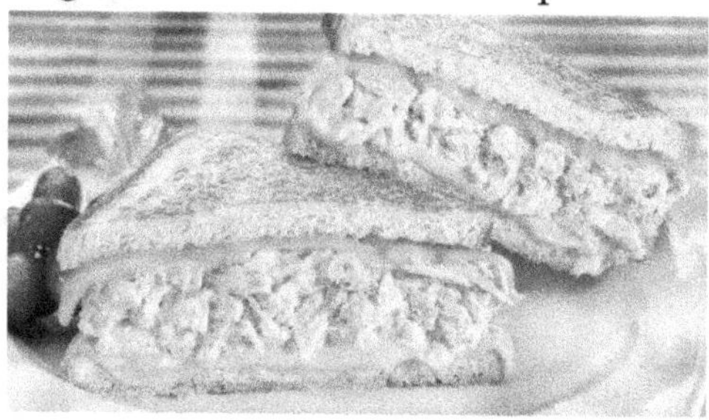

Serves: 4

Container: you will need 4 airtight containers

Time: approximately 15 minutes

Nutritional info per serving:

- Calories: 380
- Fat: 14 grams
- Protein: 21 grams
- Carbs: 36 grams

Ingredients:

- 4 slices of cheddar cheese
- 8 slices of wholegrain bread
- 1 cup corn kernels, fresh or canned
- 2 small cans of tuna (single-serve cans, half a can per sandwich)
- Salt and pepper, to taste

Method:

1. Place a slice of cheese on 4 bread slices, top with corn kernels and tuna, sprinkle with salt and pepper and then place the other slice of bread on top of each sandwich.
2. Wrap in plastic wrap to keep the sandwiches together and transfer to your airtight containers.
3. Store in the fridge until need, and place into a hot sandwich press to toast before eating!

STUFFED SWEET POTATOES

By now you should have noticed that sweet potatoes are cropping up a LOT in this recipe book! But I think they are too good not to take advantage of. These sweet potatoes are stuffed with scallions, parsley, a little cottage cheese, and some baby spinach.

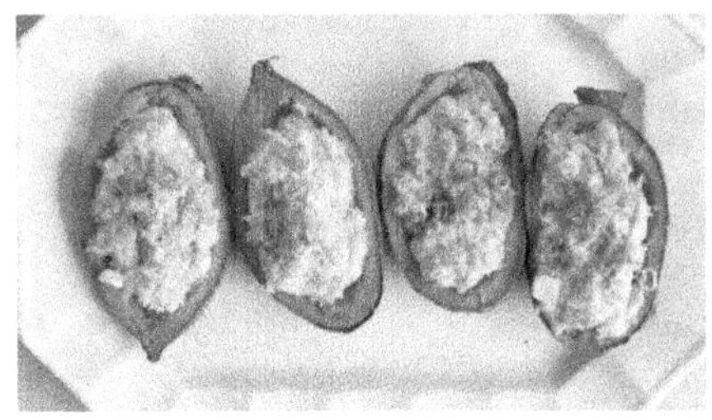

Serves: 4

Container: you will need 4 airtight containers

Time: approximately 20 minutes

Nutritional info per serving:

- Calories: 190
- Fat: 3 grams
- Protein: 9 grams
- Carbs: 27 grams

Ingredients:

- 4 sweet potatoes, pricked all over with a fork
- 1 scallion, finely chopped
- Small handful of parsley, finely chopped
- 1 cup cottage cheese
- 1 cup baby spinach leaves
- Salt and pepper, to taste

Method:

1. Introduce the sweet potatoes in the microwave and cook on HIGH for 10 minutes until they are soft all the way through.
2. Cut the sweet potatoes in half and remove the flesh with a spoon.
3. Add the potato flesh in a small bowl.
4. Add the scallions, parsley, cottage cheese, spinach, salt, and pepper, stir to combine.
5. Re-fill the sweet potatoes with the filling and place 2 halves into each of your 4 containers.
6. Place into the fridge to store until needed!

HOMEMADE HUMMUS, TOMATO, AND HAM RICE WAFER STACKS

This is a light, "snacky" lunch for the days when you feel like nibbling rather than feasting. Rice wafers, tomato, ham, and delicious homemade hummus – all with a sprinkle of salt and pepper. Delicious!

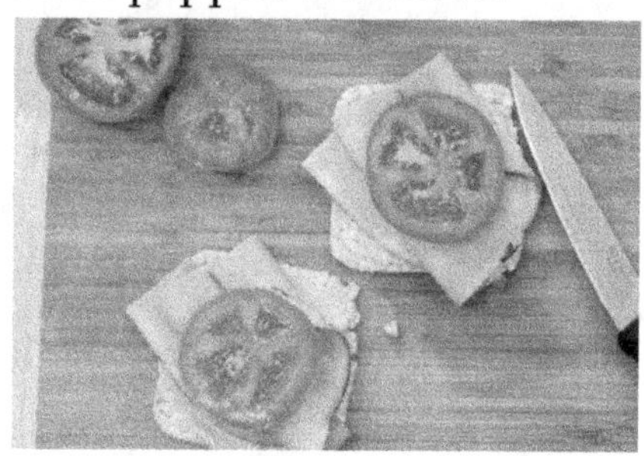

Serves: 4

Container: you will need 4 airtight containers, containers with separate compartments would be ideal!

Time: approximately 20 minutes

Nutritional info per serving:

- Calories: 340
- Fat: 19 grams
- Protein: 12 grams
- Carbs: 32 grams

Ingredients:

- 1 can of chickpeas, drained
- 1 tbsp. tahini
- 1 garlic clove
- 4 tbsp. olive oil
- 1 lemon
- Salt and pepper, to taste
- 12 rice wafers
- 2 large tomatoes, sliced
- 4 large slices of deli ham

Method:

1. Make the hummus by placing the chickpeas, tahini, garlic clove, olive oil, juice of one lemon, salt, and pepper in a blender or food processor and blending until smooth.
2. Wrap your rice wafers in plastic wrap to keep them fresh and place them into the pantry.

3. Place a good drop of hummus into one corner of your airtight containers, and then divide the tomato and ham between the containers too.

4. Cover your containers with lids and place them in the fridge until needed.

5. When it's time to pack your lunch in your work bag, simply take a container of toppings and grab a packet of wrapped rice wafers too.

6. Assemble just before eating for a fresh and crunchy lunch!

GRILLED SALMON AND SEASONAL GREENS

Fresh salmon isn't always the most affordable ingredient, but treat yourself to a few salmon lunches every few weeks. The protein and fatty acids are so worth the money spent! Use any seasonal greens you have; this recipe uses broccoli and zucchini.

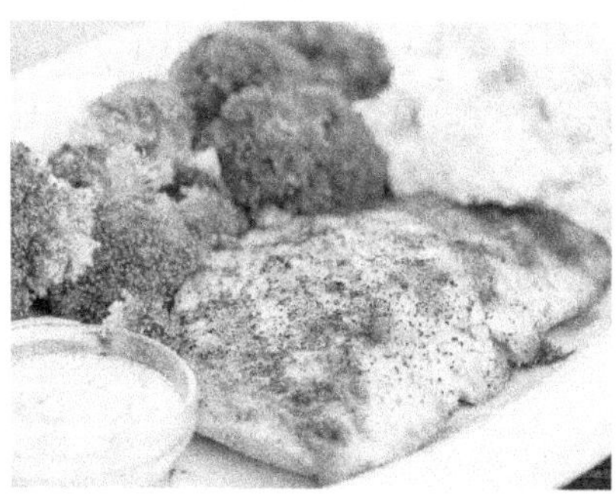

Serves: 4

Container: you will need 4 airtight containers

Time: approximately 30 minutes

Nutritional info per serving:

- Calories: 235
- Fat: 7 grams
- Protein: 30 grams
- Carbs: 13 grams

Ingredients:

- 4 small-medium salmon filets
- Salt and pepper, to taste
- Olive oil
- 1 head of broccoli, cut into florets
- 2 large zucchinis, chopped into chunks
- 1 tsp. sesame oil

Method:

1. Preheat the oven to 356 degrees Fahrenheit, then line a baking tray with a sheet of baking paper, place the salmon filets on the tray and sprinkle with salt, pepper and a little olive oil.

2. Place in the oven and bake for approximately 12-15 minutes or until cooked to your liking.

3. As the salmon cooks, prepare the greens by placing a pot of water over a high heat and bringing it to a boil, place a steaming basket or double boiler over the pot and add the greens inside, cover the basket with a lid.

4. Steam the veggies for a few minutes until just cooked, sprinkle with the sesame oil and some salt, and pepper.

5. Place one salmon filet into each container and divide the veggies between the containers.

6. Transfer the containers to the fridge to store before serving.

7. Eat hot or cold!

CHICKEN, STRAWBERRY, AND BLACK RICE SALAD

Black rice is a bit more exciting than the regular rice, and the addition of strawberries makes it even more exotic! Even though it sounds a bit strange and fancy, it's really not. Black rice is available in many supermarkets, as are strawberries in the right season! Grilled chicken is gently seasoned with lemon, salt and pepper.

Serves: 4

Container: you will need 4 airtight containers

Time: approximately 40 minutes

Nutritional info per serving:

- Calories: 380
- Fat: 3 grams
- Protein: 14 grams
- Carbs: 68 grams

Ingredients:

- 2 cups dry black rice
- 1 large chicken breast
- Olive oil
- Salt and pepper, to taste
- 1 cup strawberries, stalks removed, sliced
- 1 lemon

Method:

1. Preheat the oven to 356 degrees Fahrenheit, and then line a baking tray with baking paper.
2. Add the rice in a pot and pour 4 cups of water and a pinch of salt, bring to a boil and then reduce the heat to a simmer, cover and let simmer until the water has evaporated and the rice is cooked.
3. While the rice is cooking, cook the chicken by placing it on the lined baking tray, drizzling with olive oil, and sprinkling with salt and pepper. Bake in the preheated oven for approximately 20 minutes or until cooked through.
4. Shred the cooked chicken breast and add to the pot with the cooked black rice.
5. Add the strawberries to the pot and squeeze in the juice of one lemon.

6. Season with salt and pepper before stirring to combine.

7. Divide between 4 containers, cover and store in the fridge until needed!

SMOKED SALMON AND AVOCADO WHOLEGRAIN WRAPS

Smoked salmon and avocado, wrapped in a soft and healthy wholegrain wrap, with lots of crispy lettuce and a drizzle of vinegar dressing – all you need for a healthy lunch.

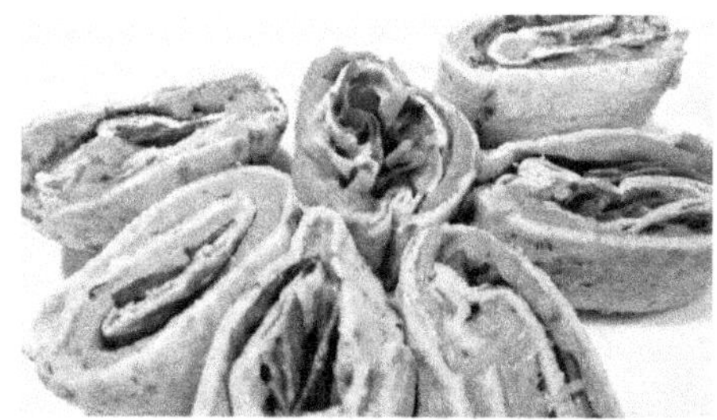

Serves: 4

Container: you will need 4 airtight containers

Time: approximately 20 minutes

Nutritional info per serving:

- Calories: 365
- Fat: 20 grams
- Protein: 10 grams
- Carbs: 37 grams

Ingredients:

- 4 wholegrain wraps
- 2 cups lettuce, roughly sliced
- 2 avocadoes, flesh sliced
- 3 oz. smoked salmon
- Olive oil
- 1 tbsp. balsamic vinegar mixed with 1 tablespoon of olive oil

Method:

1. Place your wraps on a large cutting board.
2. Add a pile of lettuce on each wrap, then add ½ avocado (sliced) on top, place the salmon on top of the avocado and drizzle with olive oil and vinegar.
3. Carefully wrap your wraps into tight parcels, transfer in your containers and store in the fridge until needed.

COLD TUNA AND PASTA SALAD

There's only a small amount of whole-grain pasta in this recipe, just enough to fill you up! Tuna, avocado, carrot, corn and bell peppers bulk-out the veggie quota for this yummy cold salad.

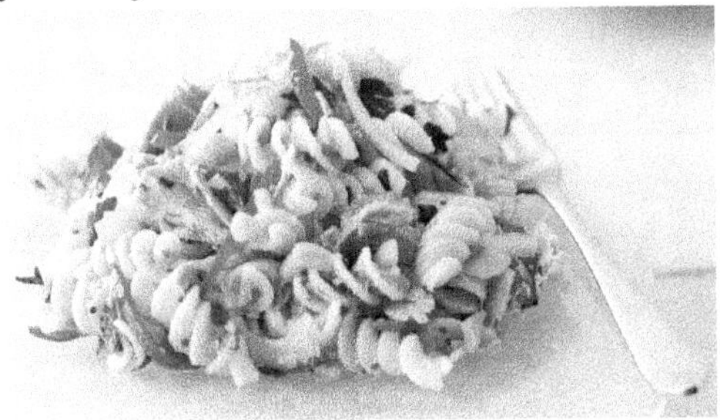

Serves: 4

Container: you will need 4 airtight containers

Time: approximately 30 minutes

Nutritional info per serving:

- Calories: 235
- Fat: 10 grams
- Protein: 10 grams
- Carbs: 28 grams

Ingredients:

- 1 ½ cups wholegrain penne pasta (or any other shape you have on hand!)
- 2 cans tuna (the single-serve cans) drained
- 2 carrots, peeled and cut into small pieces
- ¾ cup corn kernels
- 1 avocado, flesh cut into chunks
- 1 red bell pepper, core and seeds removed, flesh cut into small pieces
- Salt and pepper, to taste

Method:

1. Bring a pot of water to a boil and add pinch of salt and the dry pasta, cook until the pasta is al dente (some pastas differ so use the instructions on the package).
2. Drain the pasta and leave to cool slightly before adding the tuna, carrots, corn, avocado, bell pepper, salt, pepper, and a drizzle of olive oil.
3. Divide the pasta salad between 4 containers, cover and place in the fridge to store until needed.

4. Serve cold!

CAULIFLOWER RICE AND CHILI CHICKEN

Cauliflower rice is an angel-sent food for anyone wanting to lower their carb intake. It's affordable, easy, tasty, and low in calories. Chicken rubbed with chili and olive oil, baked in the oven to moist perfection is a pure delight to eat in between your busy work day!

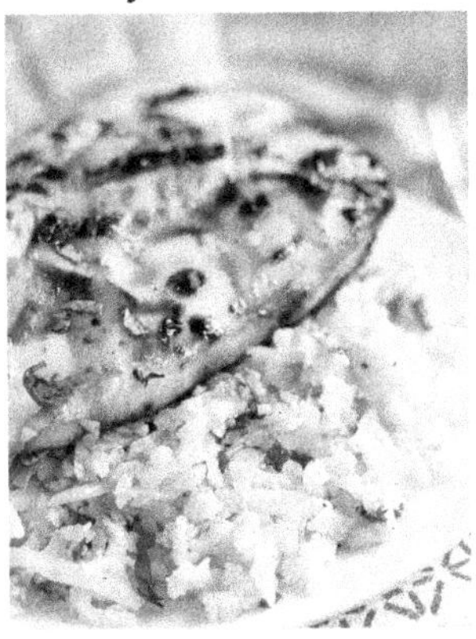

Serves: 4

Container: you will need 4 airtight containers

Time: approximately 30 minutes

Nutritional info per serving:

- Calories: 310
- Fat: 21 grams
- Protein: 21 grams
- Carbs: 12 grams

Ingredients:

- 1 head of cauliflower, core removed, florets cut into chunks
- Salt and pepper, to taste
- 4 boneless, skinless chicken thighs
- 2 tbsp. olive oil
- 1 fresh red chili, finely chopped
- 1 garlic clove, crushed
- 1 lemon, cut into quarters

Method:

1. Preheat the oven to 356 degrees Fahrenheit, and then line a baking tray with baking paper.
2. Add the cauliflower in a food processor and blend until it resembles the size and consistency of rice.
3. Transfer the cauliflower to a bowl and sprinkle with salt and pepper, place in the microwave and cook on HIGH for 5 minutes until cooked through.

4. Place the chicken thighs on the lined baking tray and sprinkle the olive oil, chili, garlic, salt and pepper on top rub to combine and make sure the chicken is well-coated.

5. Introduce the chicken into the preheated oven and bake for approximately 20 minutes or until the chicken is cooked through.

6. Divide the cauliflower rice between the 4 containers and place a chicken thigh into each container on top of the "rice".

7. Place a lemon quarter into each container, cover and place into the fridge until needed!

LOADED BROCCOLI SALAD WITH TOASTED SEEDS

More broccoli! As you can see, I use broccoli in a huge portion of my meals. The fiber, nutrients and vitamins the broccoli provides is potently perfect. Toasted seeds, red onion, and Parmesan cheese add a unique twist to this green and glorious salad.

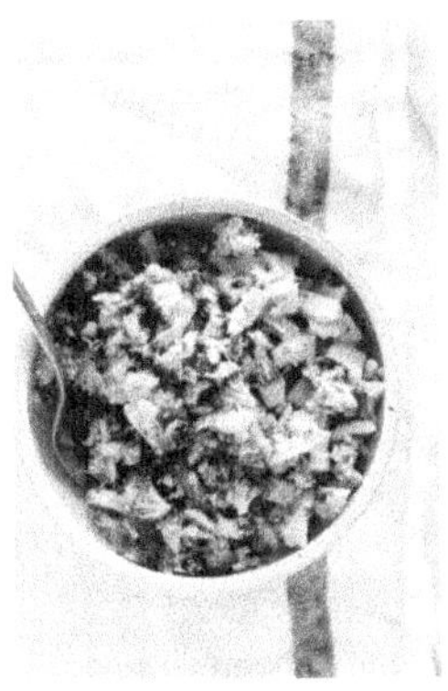

Serves: 4

Container: you will need 4 airtight containers

Time: approximately 20 minutes

Nutritional info per serving:

- Calories: 195
- Fat: 14 grams
- Protein: 11 grams
- Carbs: 12 grams

Ingredients:

- Olive oil
- 1 large head of broccoli, stalks removed, cut into florets
- ¼ red onion, finely chopped
- 2 tbsp. pumpkin seeds
- 2 tbsp. sunflower seeds
- 3 tbsp. grated Parmesan cheese
- Salt and pepper, to taste

Method:

1. Pour some olive oil in a frying pan and heat it over medium heat.
2. Add the broccoli and sauté for a few minutes.
3. Pour a few tablespoons of water into the pan and immediately cover the pan with a lid to trap the steam, this will steam the broccoli.
4. Once the water has evaporated and the broccoli is cooked but still has a "bite", add the red onion, pumpkin seeds and sunflower

seeds, continue cooking for about 1 minute until the seeds are gently toasted.

5. Divide the broccoli mixture between 4 containers and sprinkle the Parmesan over each one.

6. Finish with a sprinkle of salt and pepper and a little drizzle of olive oil.

7. Cover and place into the fridge until needed!

WHITE BEAN AND TOMATO SALAD WITH BALSAMIC DRESSING

This salad reminds me of a sundrenched afternoon in Italy. Beans should never be overlooked, they are a dieter's best friend, in my humble opinion. Gluten-free, filling, fibrous and can be put into many different dishes, beans are the best! This salad utilizes white beans, fresh tomatoes, basil and balsamic vinegar.

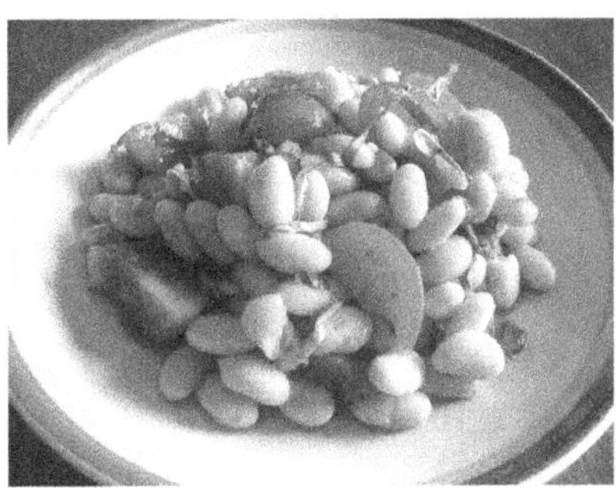

Serves: 4

Container: you will need 4 airtight containers

Time: approximately 10 minutes

Nutritional info per serving:

- Calories: 250
- Fat: 7 grams
- Protein: 13 grams
- Carbs: 33 grams

Ingredients:

- 2 cans white beans, drained
- 3 ripe tomatoes, cut into chunks
- Small handful of fresh basil, roughly chopped
- 2 tbsp. balsamic vinegar mixed with 2 tablespoons of olive oil
- Salt and pepper, to taste

Method:

1. Place the beans, tomatoes, basil, balsamic, olive oil, salt, and pepper into a small bowl and mix to combine.
2. Divide between 4 containers, cover and place into the fridge to store until needed.
3. Eat cold!

BASIL, TOMATO AND HALOUMI SALAD WITH COS AND CUCUMBER

Another recipe with basil and tomato, the combination is so tasty it should be enjoyed as often as possible. Salty haloumi cheese satisfies the palate, while lettuce and cucumber refresh and nourish you.

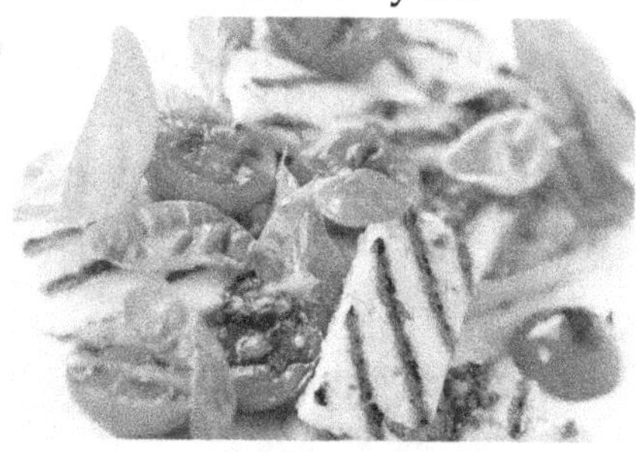

Serves: 4

Container: you will need 4 airtight containers

Time: approximately 20 minutes

Nutritional info per serving:

- Calories: 250
- Fat: 20 grams
- Protein: 11 grams
- Carbs: 8 grams

Ingredients:

- 7 oz. halloumi cheese, sliced into 12 slices
- 2 cos or Romaine lettuces, roughly chopped
- 1 cup chopped cucumber
- 3 large tomatoes, sliced
- Large handful of fresh basil, roughly chopped
- 2 tbsp. apple cider vinegar mixed with 2 tbsp. olive oil

Method:

1. Heat a non-stick frying pan over a high heat.
2. Add the halloumi slices to the pan and cook on both sides until golden.
3. Divide the lettuce, cucumber, tomatoes, basil, and halloumi between the 4 containers.
4. Sprinkle with salt and pepper, and the oil/vinegar mixture, gently toss to combine and coat with dressing.
5. Cover and place into the fridge to store until needed.

PREPPED TOPPING PACKS FOR RICE WAFERS

A variety of toppings for rice wafers, neatly packed away in a container until you're ready to DIY your rice wafers for a tasty and healthy lunch. The nutritional information includes all of the toppings plus 4 plain rice wafers. I LOVE to spread peanut butter on rice wafers and then slice quarter of a banana on top for a savory-sweet treat.

Serves: 4

Container: you will need 4 airtight containers, preferably with separated compartments

Time: approximately 10 minutes

Nutritional info per serving:

- Calories: 310
- Fat: 11 grams
- Protein: 19 grams
- Carbs: 36 grams

Ingredients:

- 1 cup cottage cheese
- 4 tbsp. chopped chives
- 1 fresh tomato, sliced
- 4 slices of deli ham or turkey
- 4 tbsp. peanut butter
- 1 banana, cut into 4 chunks
- (plus 4 rice wafers per lunch serving)

Method:

1. Place the cottage cheese, chives, tomato, ham or turkey, peanut butter, and banana in a container with separated compartments.
2. Cover and transfer to the fridge to store until needed.
3. Wrap the rice wafers in sealable bags or plastic wrap, or keep them in an airtight container at work to pull out whenever you need them!

MINCED LAMB MEAT BALLS WITH YOGURT AND CUCUMBER DIP

Meatballs for lunch? Yes! Lamb, yoghurt and cucumber is a refreshing and Greek-inspired combination. You can serve it with pita bread for extra carbs if you've had, or have got a big workout ahead of you!

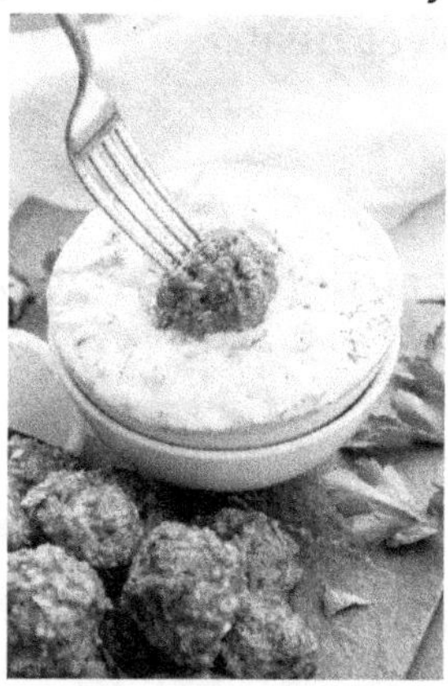

Serves: 4

Container: you will need 4 airtight containers

Time: approximately 25 minutes

Nutritional info per serving:

- Calories: 390
- Fat: 26 grams
- Protein: 31 grams
- Carbs: 4 grams

Ingredients:

- 17.5 oz. minced lamb
- ½ red onion, finely chopped
- 1 egg
- ½ cup almond flour
- Salt and pepper, to taste
- Olive oil
- ½ cup plain Greek yogurt
- ¾ cup finely chopped cucumber

Method:

1. Place the minced lamb, red onion, egg, almond flour, salt, and pepper into a bowl and stir to combine.
2. Pour some olive oil in a non-stick frying pan and heat it over medium heat.

3. Roll the lamb mixture into 16 balls and add them in 2 batches in the hot pan, cook for about 7 minutes, turning a few times until golden and cooked through.

4. Stir together the yogurt and cucumber in a small bowl.

5. Place 4 lamb balls into each container and place some yogurt mixture on top.

6. Cover and transfer to the fridge to store until needed.

7. Eat cold or hot! (Place the yogurt on the side if you want to eat the lamb balls hot, so then you don't have to heat the yogurt as well).

ONE-TRAY CHICKEN THIGH AND ROOT VEGGIE BAKED "BOWLS"

Another chicken and veggie dish! As mentioned before, you can't really go wrong with chicken and veggies when you are trying to trim down. The veggies in question here are root veggies: carrots, parsnips, beets and onions – filling, fibrous and full of minerals.

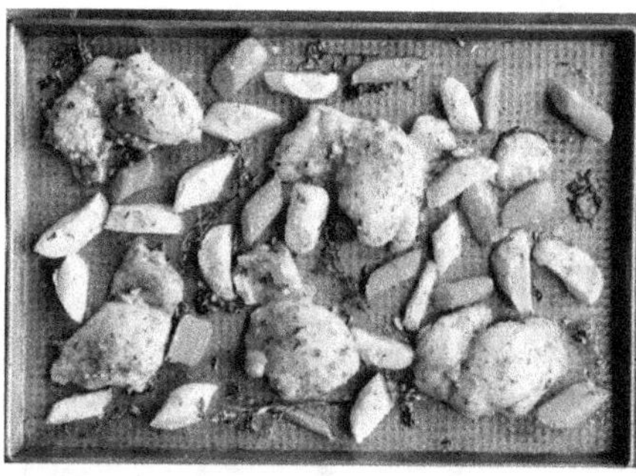

Serves: 4

Container: you will need 4 airtight containers or bowls

Time: approximately 35 minutes

Nutritional info per serving:

- Calories: 360
- Fat: 17 grams
- Protein: 29 grams
- Carbs: 23 grams

Ingredients:

- 4 boneless, skinless chicken thighs
- 2 carrots, cut into small chunks
- 2 parsnips, peeled and cut into chunks
- 2 raw beets, cut into chunks
- 1 large red onion, cut into wedges
- 1 tsp. mixed dried herbs
- Olive oil
- Salt and pepper, to taste
- 1 lemon, cut into quarters

Method:

1. Preheat the oven to 356 degrees Fahrenheit, then line a baking tray with baking paper.
2. Place the chicken thighs, carrots, parsnips, beets, onion, herbs in the tray, and a drizzle with olive oil, then add a pinch of salt and pepper and combine all of the ingredients with your hands.

3. Place the tray into the oven and bake for approximately 30 minutes or until the chicken is cooked through and the veggies are soft.
4. Divide the chicken and veggies between the 4 containers and place a lemon quarter into each container.
5. Place into the fridge to store until needed!

COLD SOBA NOODLE SALAD WITH CASHEWS, CARROT AND TOFU

Soba noodles are available at all Asian supermarkets. They are affordable, tasty, and if you get the 100% buckwheat variety, they are gluten-free. Cashews and carrot are added for flavor and crunch, and tofu for protein and flavor-soaking goodness.

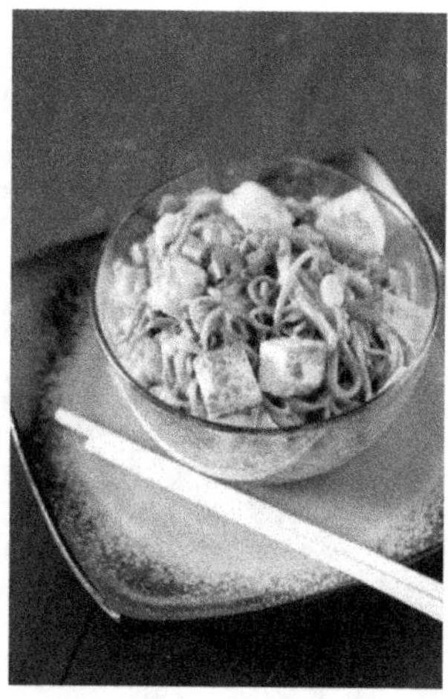

Serves: 4

Container: you will need 4 airtight containers

Time: approximately 20 minutes

Nutritional info per serving:

- Calories: 490
- Fat: 10 grams
- Protein: 22 grams
- Carbs: 87 grams

Ingredients:

- 14 oz. dry soba noodles
- 2 tbsp. sesame oil
- 2 tbsp. soy sauce
- 1 tbsp. honey
- 9 oz. firm tofu, sliced
- 1/3 cup raw cashew nuts
- 2 carrots, peeled and chopped into small pieces

Method:

1. Place a pot of water over a high heat, bring to a boil and add the soba noodles; cook until soft.
2. While the noodles are cooking, pour the sesame oil, soy sauce and honey into a small non-stick fry pan and heat it over medium heat.

3. Place the tofu slices into the hot pan and cook for a couple of minutes on each side until golden.

4. Drain the noodles and place into a bowl.

5. Add the cashews, carrots, and cooked tofu with any oil/soy sauce left in the fry pan.

6. Stir to combine.

7. Divide between the 4 containers, cover and transfer to the fridge to store until needed!

8. Best eaten cold!

DINNER

I believe that dinner time is the worst time when it comes to stress and rushing. Therefore, it's important to MEGA-prep your dinners. I'd suggest a freezer full of meals that you can whip out in the morning or the night before and leave in the fridge to thaw in time for dinner. In this section, you will find prepped pasta sauces and prepped marinated meats to store in the freezer. Marinating meat and making sauces is usually the most time-consuming part of dinner, so get the hard part out of the way well in advance!

FREEZER SOUP (PUMPKIN AND COCONUT)

Keeping a soup in the freezer, stored in single-serve containers is a very smart move indeed. This pumpkin and coconut soup freezes really well and it's filling enough to satisfy you, but light enough to enjoy during any season. Super low in calories, so you can add a piece of buttered toast and not ruin your diet (well, that's my logic anyway!).

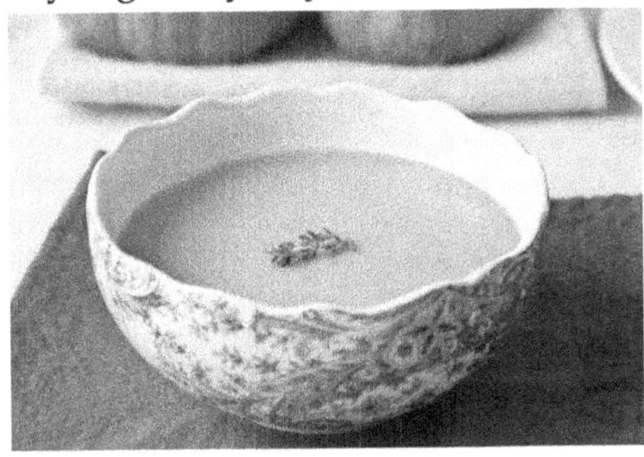

Serves: 6

Container: you will need 6 airtight, freezer-safe containers

Time: approximately 45 minutes

Nutritional info per serving:

- Calories: 105
- Fat: 4 grams
- Protein: 5 grams
- Carbs: 16 grams

Ingredients:

- 6 cups cubed pumpkin (skin removed, about 1 medium-sized pumpkin)
- 1 onion, finely chopped
- 2 carrots, cut into chunks
- 3 cups (24fl oz.) chicken stock
- Salt and pepper, to taste
- 1 cup (8fl oz.) coconut milk

Method:

1. Place the pumpkin, onion, carrots, stock, salt, and pepper in a pot and bring to a boil, reduce the heat to low and simmer covered for about 25 minutes or until the veggies are soft.
2. Using a hand-held blender, process until smooth.
3. Stir the coconut milk in the soup, taste, and add more salt and pepper if needed.

4. Allow it to cool slightly before pouring into 6 containers, covering, then packing them away into the freezer!
5. Remember to label the containers with masking tape and a sharpie so you can keep track of when the soup was made.
6. Simply take out of the freezer the morning of the day you want to have the soup for dinner, and leave to thaw in a small pot.
7. Heat up in the pot or microwave in a bowl.

SPICY LENTIL STEW WITH SWEET POTATO MASH AND CILANTRO

This is a totally Winter dream dinner dish. I recommend making some servings of this stew, mash them and keep in the freezer. Super easy, affordable, filling, and nourishing. Add as much chili as you like, according to your spice preference!

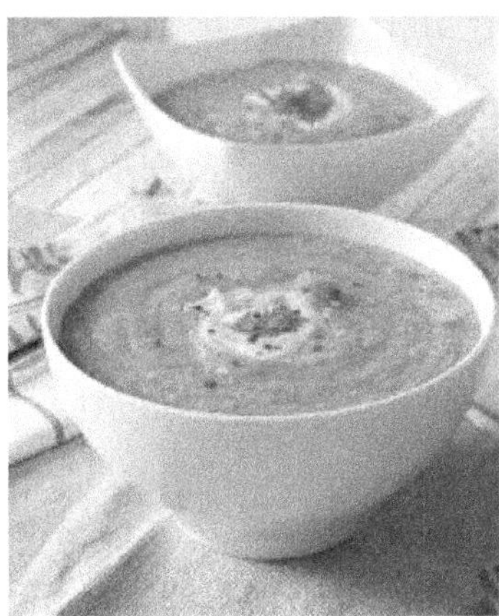

Serves: 6

Container: you will need 6 airtight containers

Time: approximately 40 minutes

Nutritional info per serving:

- Calories: 270
- Fat: 5 grams
- Protein: 19 grams
- Carbs: 34 grams

Ingredients:

- Olive oil
- 1 onion, finely chopped
- 1 tsp. cumin
- 1 tsp. chili powder
- 1 tsp. ground coriander
- 1 can (14 oz.) chopped tomatoes
- 2 cans (14 oz.) brown lentils, drained
- Salt and pepper, to taste
- 1 cup (8fl oz.) chicken stock
- 2 large sweet potatoes, cut into cubes
- Large handful of cilantro, roughly chopped

Method:

1. Pour some olive oil in a pot and heat it over medium heat.

2. Add the onion, cumin, chili, ground coriander, tomatoes, lentils, salt, and pepper; stir to combine.
3. Add the chicken stock to the pot.
4. Allow it to simmer for about 20 minutes until thick and rich.
5. As the lentil stew simmers, cook the sweet potatoes by pricking all over with a fork and cooking in the microwave on HIGH for 10 minutes until soft all the way through.
6. Cut the cooked sweet potatoes into chunks and place in a bowl (I keep the skin on, it has nutrients!), add some salt and pepper and mash with a fork.
7. Divide the sweet potato mash between 6 containers then divide the lentil stew between the containers, spooning it on top of the sweet potatoes.
8. Sprinkle with fresh cilantro, cover and place into the fridge or freezer (or both, freeze 3, fridge 3!) until needed.

RAINBOW CHICKEN SALAD

The "rainbow" comes from the beautiful array of colors in this fresh and yummy salad. Red cabbage, carrot, cucumber, yellow bell peppers, lettuce and tomatoes burst onto the plate, with tender chicken. Make a big bowl of this on your meal-prep day and eat it for dinner for 3 nights after.

Serves: 6 (enough for 3 nights for 2 people)

Container: you will need one large airtight container or 6 smaller airtight containers

Time: approximately 30 minutes

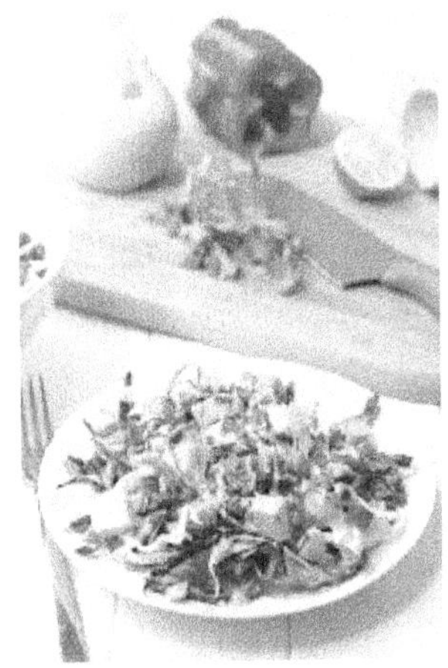

Nutritional info per serving:

- Calories: 205
- Fat: 6 grams
- Protein: 22 grams
- Carbs: 15 grams

Ingredients:

- 2 chicken breasts
- Olive oil
- Salt and pepper, to taste
- ½ head of red cabbage, thinly sliced
- 2 carrots, grated
- 1 cup cubed cucumber
- 2 yellow bell peppers, core and seeds removed, thinly sliced
- ½ head iceberg lettuce, roughly chopped
- 2 tomatoes, chopped into chunks
- 2 tbsp. balsamic vinegar mixed with 2 tbsp. olive oil

Method:

1. Preheat the oven to 356 degrees Fahrenheit, then line a baking tray with baking paper.
2. Place the chicken breasts on the tray and rub with olive oil, salt, and pepper, introduce in the oven and bake for approximately 25 minutes or until cooked all the way through.
3. Slice the cooked chicken breasts into thin slices.
4. Place the cabbage, carrot, cucumber, bell peppers, lettuce, tomatoes, balsamic vinegar, olive oil, and chicken in a large bowl and gently toss to combine and coat in oil and vinegar.
5. Divide the salad between the 6 containers, cover and transfer to the fridge to store until needed!
6. Eat within 3 nights of cooking (3 dinners for 2 people).

VEGGIE STACKS WITH FETA AND MINT

There's so much fresh mint in my garden at the moment I am finding myself adding it to so many of my recipes and meals! It goes so well with feta cheese, and just as well with veggies. These stacks feature mushrooms, zucchini, eggplant, and tomato.

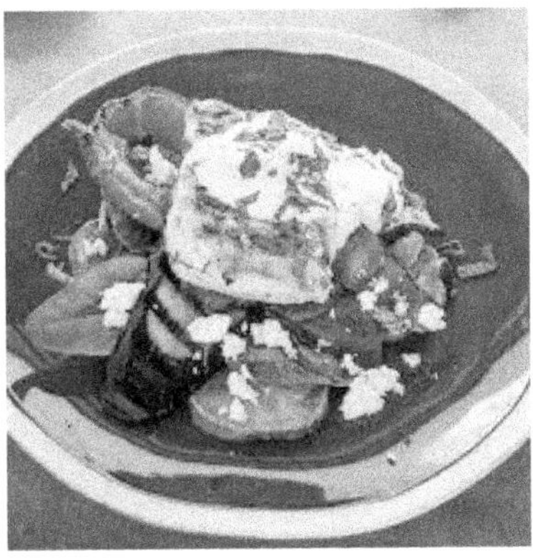

Serves: 4

Container: you will need 4 airtight containers

Time: approximately 25 minutes

Nutritional info per serving:

- Calories: 230
- Fat: 12 grams
- Protein: 10 grams
- Carbs: 18 grams

Ingredients:

- 8 large Portobello mushrooms
- 2 large zucchinis, sliced lengthways
- 1 large eggplant, sliced into 8 slices
- 2 large tomatoes, sliced
- 2 tbsp. olive oil
- 2 garlic cloves, crushed
- Salt and pepper, to taste
- 3.5 oz. feta cheese
- Small handful fresh mint leaves

Method:

1. Preheat the oven to 356 degrees Fahrenheit, then line a baking tray with baking paper.
2. Lay the mushrooms, zucchini slices, eggplant slices, and tomato slices on the tray and drizzle with the olive oil, and then add garlic, salt, and pepper.

3. Place the tray in the oven and bake for approximately 20 minutes until tender and golden.

4. Create your stacks by layering in this order: mushrooms, feta, zucchini slices, feta, eggplant slices, mint, tomato slices, feta, mint.

5. Place a skewer through the middle of each stack to keep them together if you like!

6. Pack away into your containers, cover and place in the fridge until needed.

LAMB AND RED ONION SKEWERS

These skewers have two core ingredients: lamb and red onion. You can make a big batch of these and add any salad to go with it.

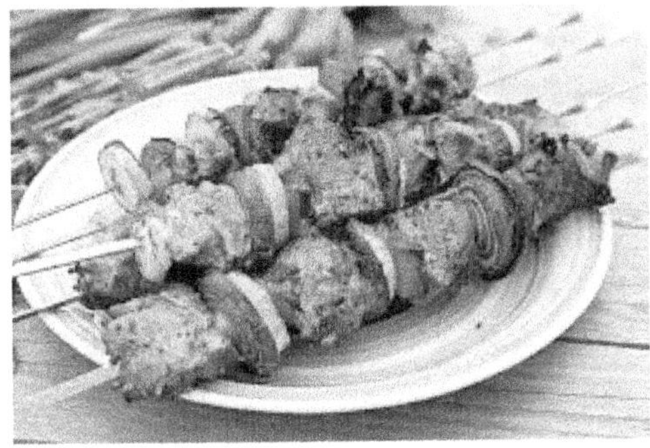

Serves: 8 skewers (2 skewers per serving, so 4 servings)

Container: store in one large, airtight container and take them out as you need them

Time: approximately 25 minutes

Nutritional info per serving:

- Calories: 270
- Fat: 19 grams
- Protein: 27 grams
- Carbs: 4 grams

Ingredients:

- 4 lamb leg steaks, cut into cubes
- 2 red onions, cut into 8 wedges each
- 2 tbsp. olive oil
- Salt and pepper, to taste
- 8 skewers

Method:

1. Preheat the oven to 400 degrees Fahrenheit, then line a baking tray with some baking paper.
2. Load the skewers by alternating the lamb and onion until full (but leave an inch on either side of the skewers so you can pick them up easily).
3. Rub the onion and lamb skewers with olive oil and sprinkle salt and pepper, and then place on the tray.
4. Place the tray into the oven and bake for approximately 20 minutes, turning once, until the onions are cooked and beginning to turn golden, and the lamb is cooked but still pink inside.

5. Leave the skewers to cool slightly before packing away in a large
    container, covering and storing in the fridge until needed.

VEGGIE BURGERS PATTIES

These veggie burger patties can be eaten with a simple salad, or turned into a delicious burger with a wholegrain bun, tomato, lettuce, relish, and mustard. The nutritional information provided is for the patties only. These patties are cooked in the oven which eliminates the need for oil, and therefore, brings fewer calories.

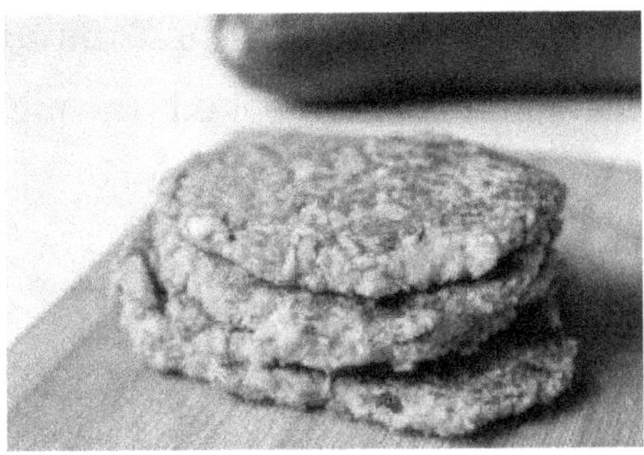

Serves: makes 8 large patties

Container: store in one airtight container and take them out as you need them, you can also freeze them too, wrap them individually in greaseproof paper so they don't stick together in the container

Time: approximately 25 minutes

Nutritional info per serving: Per patty

- Calories: 130
- Fat: 4 grams
- Protein: 7 grams
- Carbs: 14 grams

Ingredients:

- 5 Portobello mushrooms, cut into small pieces
- 1 cup corn kernels
- 1 cup chickpeas, drained and rinsed
- 2 eggs, lightly beaten
- 1 cup almond flour
- Large handful of fresh parsley, finely chopped
- 1 tsp. ground cumin
- 1 tsp. ground coriander
- 1 tsp. chili powder
- Salt and pepper, to taste

Method:

1. Preheat the oven to 356 degrees Fahrenheit, then line a baking tray with baking paper.

2. Place all ingredients into a large bowl and add a pinch of salt and pepper.
3. Vigorously stir until thoroughly combined.
4. Shape the mixture into 8 large patties.
5. Place the patties on the baking tray and introduce into the oven.
6. Bake for about 7 minutes on each side (just take the tray out of the oven and turn the patties over after 7 minutes then put them back in for another 7) or until cooked through and golden on the outside.
7. Stack into an airtight container and store in the fridge until needed.

MEXICAN-INSPIRED SHEPHERD'S PIE

Black beans, cilantro, chili, and sweet potatoes make up the bulk of this yummy shepherd's pie with a Mexican twist. Make a big dish of it, cut it into servings, and throw it in the fridge or freezer for dinners all week long!

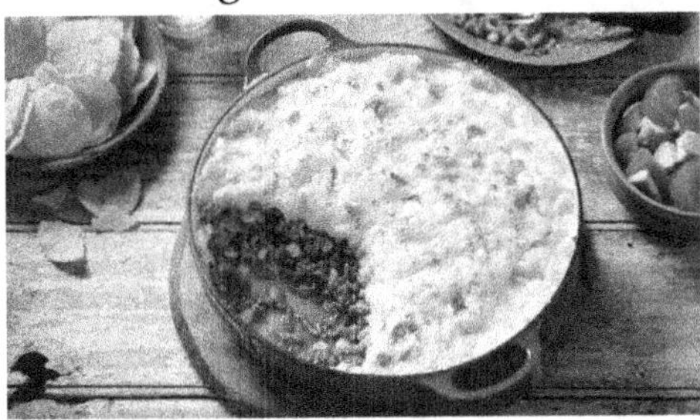

Serves: 1 large pie with 8 servings

Container: store in one large container or 8 single-serve containers if freezing for single portions

Time: approximately 45 minutes

Nutritional info per serving:

- Calories: 210
- Fat: 5 grams
- Protein: 18 grams
- Carbs: 21 grams

Ingredients:

- Olive oil
- 1 onion, finely chopped
- 17 oz. minced beef
- 2 cans (14 oz.) black beans, drained
- 1 tsp. chili powder
- 1 tsp. coriander
- 1 can (14 oz.) chopped tomatoes
- 2 large sweet potatoes, chopped into chunks
- Salt and pepper, to taste
- Large handful cilantro, roughly chopped

Method:

1. Preheat to oven to 356 degrees Fahrenheit.
2. Drizzle some olive oil into a large pot and heat it over medium heat.
3. Add the onions to the pot and sauté until soft.
4. Add the minced beef and sauté until browned.

5. Add the black beans, chili powder, coriander, and canned tomatoes, stir to combine.
6. Leave to simmer for about 10 minutes as you prepare the sweet potatoes.
7. Prick the sweet potatoes all over and place into the microwave, cook on HIGH for 10 minutes until soft all the way through.
8. Cut the sweet potatoes into chunks and place in a bowl. Mash with a potato masher or fork, add a pinch of salt and pepper and stir through.
9. Pour the mince and bean mixture into a large baking dish and spread the mashed sweet potatoes on top.
10. Sprinkle the coriander on top of the sweet potatoes.
11. Place into the oven and bake for approximately 30 minutes until golden.
12. Leave to cool before cutting into 8 pieces, stacking in your airtight container/and storing in the fridge or freezer until needed.

SWISS CHARD AND RICOTTA CRUST-LESS PIE

Swiss chard, ricotta, eggs, and a little bit of grated cheddar are the key ingredients in this protein-heavy, carb-light pie. Because there's no crust or pastry base, this is really more like a quiche, but "pie" always sounds better to me! Because it's very low in calories, you can serve it with a robust green salad with added nuts and seeds, and perhaps some roasted root veggies. Ideal for dinners on nights where you don't want to, or shouldn't go for a full-on, heavy meal.

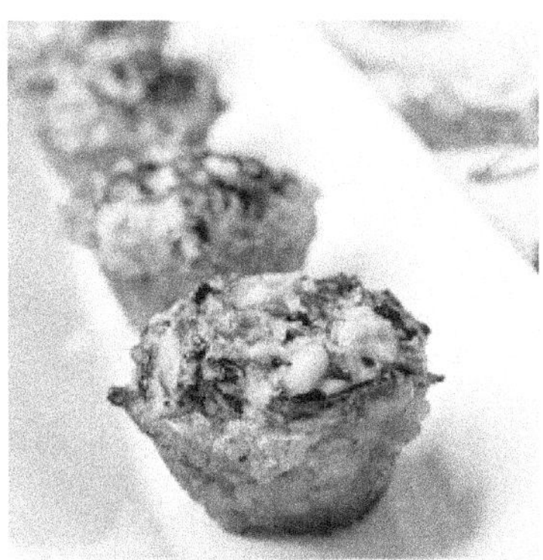

Serves: 6 slices

Container: you will need 1 large container or 6 small ones if storing or freezing individually. If storing in 1 large, separate the slices with greaseproof paper so they don't stick together.

Time: approximately 30 minutes

Nutritional info per serving:

- Calories: 200
- Fat: 14 grams
- Protein: 14 grams
- Carbs: 4 grams

Ingredients:

- Butter or cooking oil spray
- 5 eggs
- 9 oz. ricotta cheese
- 4 cups shredded Swiss chard
- 1 onion, finely chopped
- ½ cup grated cheddar cheese
- Handful of fresh parsley, finely chopped
- ½tsp baking powder
- Salt and pepper, to taste

Method:

1. Preheat the oven to 356 degrees Fahrenheit, and grease a baking dish with butter or cooking oil spray.
2. Place all the ingredients, plus a pinch of salt and pepper in a bowl and whisk until fully combined.
3. Pour in your prepared baking dish and place into the oven.
4. Bake for approximately 25 minutes or until just set and beginning to turn golden on top.
5. Slice into 6 pieces, pack into your chosen containers, cover and store in the fridge or freezer until needed!
6. A small drop of tomato relish goes really well on the side of this crust-less pie.

STEAK AND ZOODLE SALAD

"Zoodles" are noodles made from zucchinis. They've become rather popular over the last few years, as they have barely any calories but still resemble the look, texture and flavor-carrying abilities of noodles. Strips of steak, sprinkles of sesame seeds, and a lemony-olive oil dressing- ideal for both dinner and lunch!

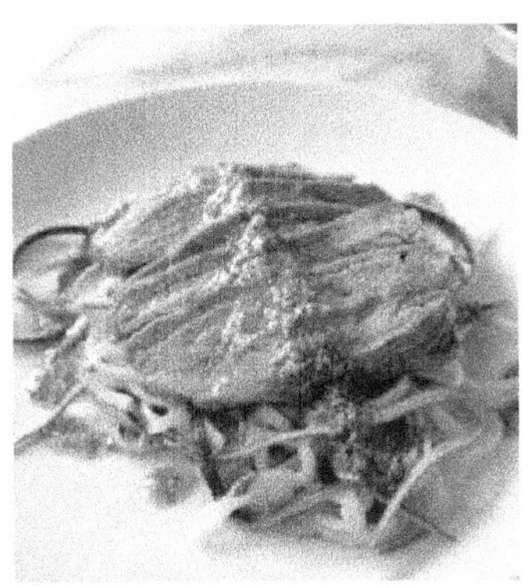

Serves: 4

Container: you will need 4 airtight containers, or 1 large container

Time: approximately 25 minutes

Nutritional info per serving:

- Calories: 365
- Fat: 22 grams
- Protein: 36 grams
- Carbs: 7 grams

Ingredients:

- 3 large zucchinis, cut into noodles using a spiralizer
- Salt and pepper, to taste
- Olive oil
- 2 sirloin steaks (or 1 really large one, use your judgment to figure out how much steak you'd like for each serving)
- Juice of one lemon mixed with 2 tbsp. of olive oil
- 2 tbsp. sesame seeds

Method:

1. Place the zucchini noodles in a microwave-safe bowl and cook in the microwave for 1 minute. Don't overcook them, as you don't want them to be slushy or mushy! Sprinkle with salt and pepper and set aside.

2. Heat a small amount of olive oil in a non-stick frying pan.

3. Place your steak in the hot frying pan and cook to your liking. The transfer to the cutting board to rest. You can season the steak with salt and pepper at this stage.

4. Keep the pan on the heat and add the sesame seeds to the pan and toast them in the leftover steak juices until golden and fragrant.

5. Thinly slice your steak and add to the bowl with the zoodles, then add the sesame seeds and the olive oil and lemon dressing, stir to combine.

6. Pack away into your container/s, cover and place in the fridge to store until needed!

7. I love to eat this meal cold, right out of the fridge.

STIR-FRIED BROWN RICE WITH CHICKEN AND VEGGIE JEWELS

I call the veggies used in this dish "jewels" because they are cut into little squares and their glossy red, green and orange colors shine amongst the earthy brown rice and chicken. And sometimes, it's just more fun to give a dish a romantic name!

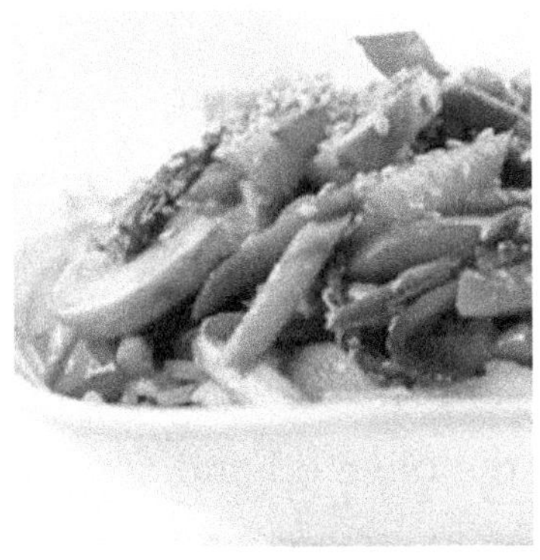

Serves: 4

Container: you will need 4 airtight containers

Time: approximately 35 minutes

Nutritional info per serving:

- Calories: 420
- Fat: 12 grams
- Protein: 21 grams
- Carbs: 61 grams

Ingredients:

- 2 large chicken breasts
- Olive oil
- Salt and pepper
- 1 tsp. chili flakes
- 1 ½ cups dry brown rice
- 1 garlic clove, crushed
- 2 red bell peppers, core and seeds removed, cut into small pieces
- 2 scallions, finely chopped
- 8 spears of asparagus, cut into small pieces (the same size as the bell pepper pieces)
- 2 carrots, peeled and cut into pieces to match the asparagus and bell pepper pieces
- 2 tbsp. olive oil mixed with 1 tbsp. soy sauce

Method:

1. Preheat the oven to 356 degrees Fahrenheit, then line a baking tray with baking paper.
2. Place the chicken breasts on the tray and drizzle with olive oil, salt, pepper, and chili flakes. Then place into the oven for approximately 20 minutes or until the chicken is cooked through.
3. Leave the chicken to rest for a few minutes before cutting into small pieces.
4. Cook the rice while the chicken is cooking: place the brown rice into a pot and add 2 cups of water, place over high heat and bring to a boil, then reduce to a simmer and cook with the lid on until the water has evaporated and the rice is cooked.
5. Add the garlic, peppers, scallions, asparagus, and carrot to the pot of rice and add the olive oil and soy sauce mixture; turn the heat up to high and keep stirring as the veggies cook in the rice – you can use a wok or fry pan for this step, but I just use the pot the rice cooked in to save myself from another dish to wash up! It works perfectly well.
6. Add the chopped cooked chicken to the pot, stir through and leave to cool before dividing between your containers. Cover and store in the fridge or freezer until needed!

PREPPED QUINOA SUSHI ROLLS

Quinoa is a healthy substitute for the regular sushi rice. These sushi rolls don't contain any meat, so they are fine to be left in the fridge for a few days and feasted on as a light dinner. Tofu, veggies, quinoa, nori and sesame seeds – fresh and tasty!

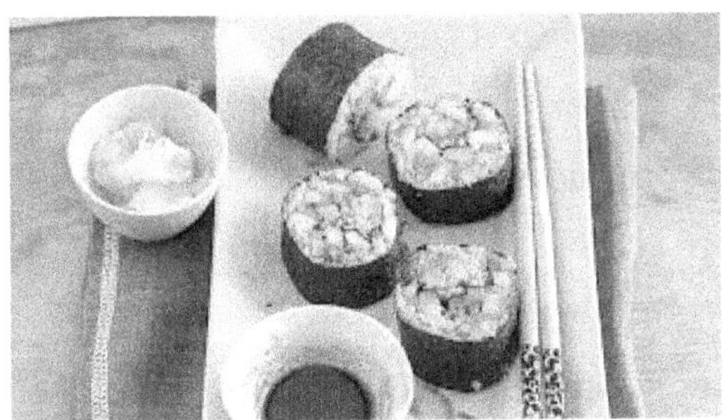

Serves: 6 sushi rolls (about 1 roll per serving)

Container: you will need 1 large container

Time: approximately 25 minutes

Nutritional info per serving:

- Calories: 280
- Fat: 9 grams
- Protein: 18 grams
- Carbs: 29 grams

Ingredients:

- 1 cup quinoa
- 1 ½ cups water
- 14 oz. firm tofu, cut into strips
- 2 tbsp. soy sauce
- 1 tsp. sesame oil
- 1 tbsp. honey
- 6 nori sheets (sushi seaweed)
- 2 tbsp. sesame seeds, lightly toasted in a dry fry pan
- 1 red bell pepper, core and seeds removed, sliced
- 1 carrot, peeled and sliced into thin strips

Method:

1. Thoroughly rinse the quinoa in a sieve to remove the bitter outer layer.
2. Bring a small pot of water to a boil and add the quinoa, stir to combine, then turn the heat down to a simmer, cover, and cook for 12-15 minutes or until the liquid has evaporated and the quinoa is soft.

3. While the quinoa is cooking, prepare the tofu: place the soy sauce, sesame oil, honey, and tofu into a small frying pan over a medium heat, cook for a few minutes until golden and cooked-through, set aside.
4. Lay the nori sheets on a large cutting board, have your tofu, cooked quinoa, toasted sesame seeds, and sliced veggies close by.
5. Spread a thin layer of quinoa onto each nori sheet, leaving an inch-wide gap at the top of each sheet.
6. Lay the tofu, carrot and bell peppers in a line in the center of the nori sheet (horizontally).
7. Sprinkle the sesame seeds on top of the tofu and veggies on each nori sheet.
8. Tightly roll the sushi and seal the ends with warm water.
9. Don't slice yet, wait until you're ready to eat to slice just before eating.
10. Pack the sushi rolls into your container and store in the fridge until needed!

Tender white fish, coated in beaten egg and crispy bread crumbs makes up for a perfect dinner anytime. Pop into the freezer and pull out whenever you want a tasty and highly-nutritious dinner! Serve with boiled potatoes and peas for a classic, British-inspired supper, or put in a taco or burger for a comfort food twist.

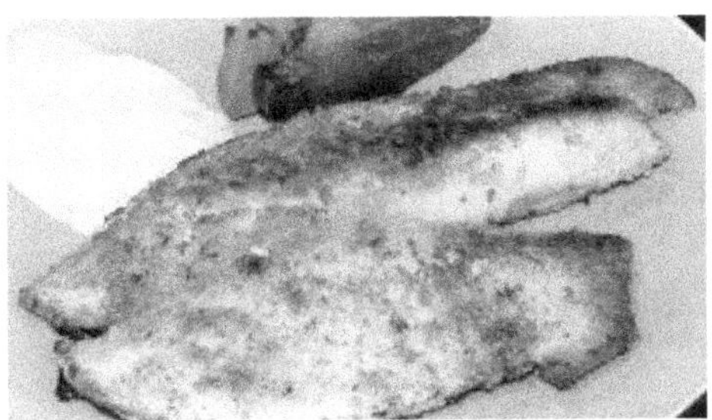

Serves: 12 breaded fish pieces (from 4 fillets, I would say 6 servings in total)

Container: you will need a small airtight container with greaseproof paper to separate the layers of fish so they don't stick together in the freezer.

Time: approximately 15 minutes

Nutritional info per serving:

- Calories: 190
- Fat: 5 grams
- Protein: 25 grams
- Carbs: 17 grams

Ingredients:

- 2 eggs, lightly beaten
- 1 cup breadcrumbs mixed with a pinch of salt and pepper
- 4 large white fish filets, cut into 3 pieces each

Method:

1. Prepare by setting the working space by beating the egg in a small bowl, and mixing the breadcrumbs with salt and pepper spread in a plate, then have your fish pieces next to them on a plate, ready to be dipped.
2. Have a tray lined with a sheet of baking paper ready too, so you can put the coated fish on it to freeze.
3. Dip the fish pieces in the beaten eggs and transfer them straight into the breadcrumbs, turning to coat thoroughly on all sides.
4. Place the coated fish on your lined tray, cover with plastic wrap and place into the freezer until almost frozen.

5. Place the almost-frozen fish pieces in a small container lined with baking paper, place another layer of paper between each layer of fish so they don't stick together.

6. Place straight into the oven from the freezer when you want to eat them! Don't thaw them out first.

GREEN BEAN, POTATO, AND PEA CURRY

If you skip the rice, this curry is actually very light, despite the decent dose of potatoes! Green beans, peas and coconut milk infused with quality store-bought green curry paste and garnished with cilantro and red chili for a special and satisfying meal - this curry is fantastic and can be stored well in the freezer too.

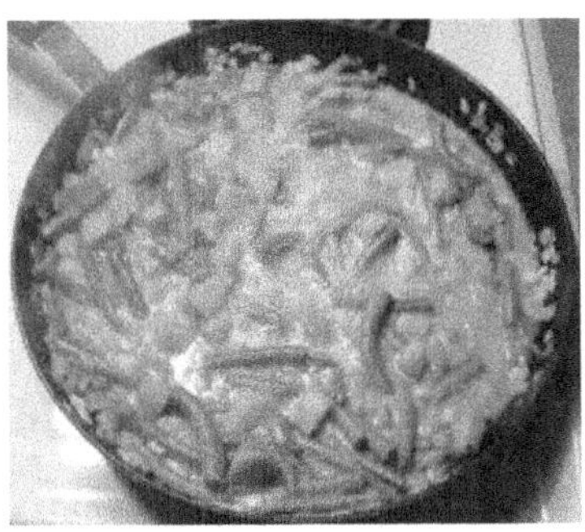

Serves: 6

Container: you will need 6 airtight containers

Time: approximately 30 minutes

Nutritional info per serving:

- Calories: 460
- Fat: 26 grams
- Protein: 11 grams
- Carbs: 47 grams

Ingredients:

- Olive oil
- 4 garlic cloves, finely chopped
- 1 onion, finely chopped
- 4 tbsp. store-bought green curry paste
- 5 large potatoes, cut into cubes or chunks
- 2 cups frozen green beans
- 2 cups frozen peas
- 1 cup (8fl oz.) chicken or vegetable broth
- 3 cups (24fl oz.) coconut milk
- Salt, to taste

Method:

1. Drizzle some olive oil into a large pot or pan and heat it over a medium heat.
2. Add the garlic, onions, and curry paste, stir to combine and leave to sauté for a couple of minutes until the curry paste is fragrant.

3. Add the potatoes, beans, peas, broth, and coconut milk to the pot and stir to combine, add a pinch of salt to season.

4. Allow the curry to boil for approximately 20 minutes or until the potatoes are soft but not mushy.

5. Leave to cool before dividing between 6 containers, covering and placing into the fridge or freezer.

COCONUT-POACHED FISH WITH PEANUTS AND ASIAN GREENS

White fish, lightly poached in coconut milk, sprinkled with peanuts and served on a bed of steamed bok choy - this dish might sound complex, but it's really so simple and wholesome. For some extra energy, serve with brown rice.

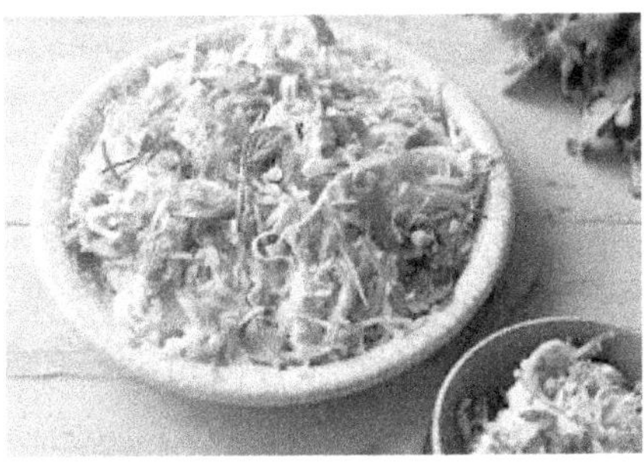

Serves: 4

Container: you will need 4 airtight containers

Time: approximately 25 minutes

Nutritional info per serving:

- Calories: 440
- Fat: 32 grams
- Protein: 42 grams
- Carbs: 10 grams

Ingredients:

- 1 ½ cups (12fl oz.) coconut milk
- 1 tsp. soy sauce
- 1 tsp. fish sauce
- 1 tsp. chili flakes
- 4 white fish filets
- 2 bunches of bok choy, base removed, leaves washed
- ½ cup roasted, salted peanuts
- 1 tsp. sesame oil

Method:

1. Add the coconut milk, soy sauce, fish sauce, chili flakes, and fish filets in a deep frying pan or pot and heat over medium heat.
2. Bring to a gentle boil and leave to simmer for about 10 minutes or until the fish is just cooked.
3. Add the bokchoi to the pot and cover the pot with the lid, leave for 1 minute to gently steam the bok choy.

4. Divide the fish, bok choy, and coconut milk between 4 containers and sprinkle the peanuts and sesame oil over the top, cover and place into the fridge or freezer to store until needed.

5. If you like, a sprinkle of fresh chili and cilantro is a gorgeous addition before eating.

TACO FREEZER PACKETS

These packets are just like the smoothie packets back in the Breakfast section, but they are for tacos! Chicken, bell peppers, onion, spices, and tomatoes all packed into sealable bags and stashed in the freezer. Simply leave them out to thaw then throw the contents into a hot fry pan to cook, then load in a tortilla, add some guacamole and you're good to go!

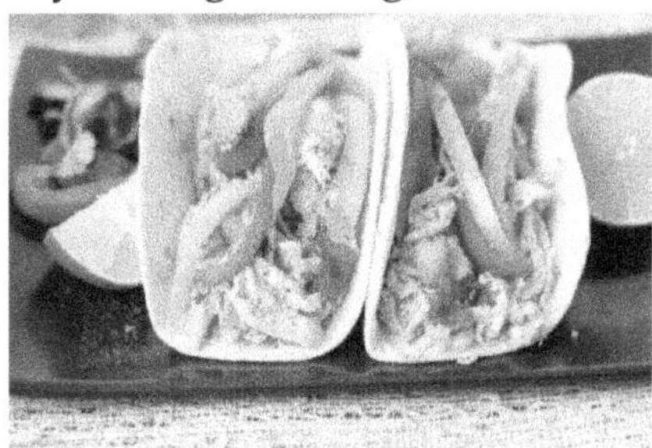

Serves: 8 packets (1 packet per serving)

Container: you will need 8 freezer-friendly, sealable bags

Time: approximately 15 minutes

Nutritional info per serving:

- Calories: 170
- Fat: 5 grams
- Protein: 20 grams
- Carbs: 12 grams

Ingredients:

- 3 large chicken breasts, cut into small slices
- 3 red bell peppers, core and seeds removed, thinly sliced
- 2 red onions, thinly sliced
- 2 cans (14 oz.) chopped tomatoes
- 6 garlic cloves, finely chopped
- 2 tsp. paprika
- 1 tsp. ground cumin
- 1 tsp. ground coriander
- 1 tsp. chili powder
- 2 tbsp. olive oil

Method:

1. Place all the ingredients in a large bowl and stir to combine, making sure every piece of chicken and vegetables is coated in olive oil and spices.
2. Divide the mixture between 8 freezer-safe sealable bags, seal and stack into the fridge to store until needed.

3. Leave to thaw before sautéing in a hot frying pan until cooked all the way through and the onions and bell peppers are slightly charred.

These freezer packets feature breaded chicken, which you can place on a baking tray and bake in the oven, straight from the freezer. Great for chicken and veggie tray bakes with any veggies you like! You'll thank yourself for prepping these protein-filled packets!

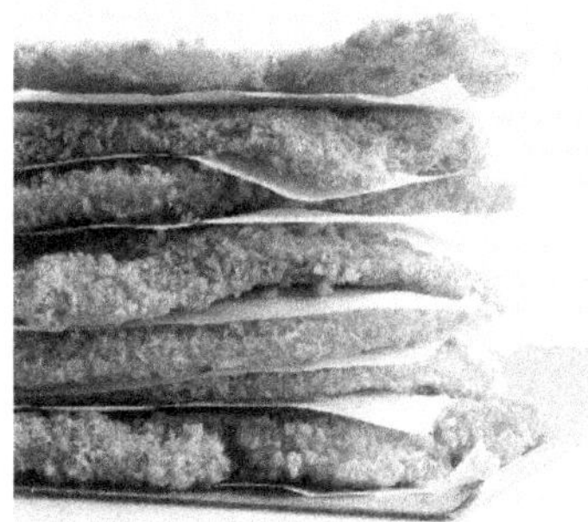

Serves: 8 freezer packets, each with 3 small pieces of chicken (1 serving per packet)

Container: you will need 8 freezer-friendly, sealable bags

Time: approximately 15 minutes

Nutritional info per serving:

- Calories: 265
- Fat: 3 grams
- Protein: 35 grams
- Carbs: 22 grams

Ingredients:

- 2 eggs, lightly beaten
- 2 cups breadcrumbs mixed with a pinch of salt and pepper
- 4 large chicken breasts, each cut into 6 pieces

Method:

1. Prepare your workspace by beating the eggs in a small bowl next to a plate of breadcrumbs mixed with salt and pepper.
2. Line a baking tray with baking paper and keep nearby so you can place your breaded chicken on it.
3. Take your chicken pieces and dip them in the egg, then straight into the breadcrumbs, turning a few times to thoroughly coat in breadcrumbs.
4. Place the breaded chicken pieces on your lined tray, cover in plastic wrap and place in the freezer.
5. Once frozen, divide the chicken pieces between 8 freezer bags and stack into the freezer to store until needed!

6. To cook, simply preheat your oven to 356 degrees Fahrenheit, place the chicken pieces on a lined baking tray and bake for about 25 minutes or until cooked through, no need to thaw first.

MARINATED STEAK FREEZER PACKETS

Next in the freezer packet series is the marinated steak. Tender strips of beef with a tasty marinade – perfect for stir-frying with veggies and serving on a little bed of brown rice!

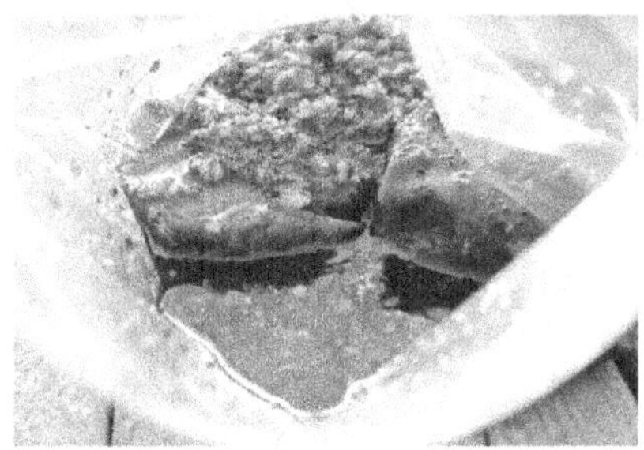

Serves: 8 packets (1 serving per packet)

Container: you will need 8 freezer-friendly, sealable bags

Time: approximately 15 minutes

Nutritional info per serving:

- Calories: 220
- Fat: 10 grams
- Protein: 28 grams
- Carbs: 2 grams

Ingredients:

- 4 beef steaks, cut into slices
- 2 tbsp. olive oil
- 2 tbsp. soy sauce
- 1 tbsp. honey
- Salt and pepper, to taste

Method:

1. Place the steak strips, olive oil, soy sauce, honey, and a pinch of salt, and pepper into a bowl and stir to combine, making sure each piece of meat is coated in oil, honey, and sauce.
2. Divide the marinated steak between 8 freezer-safe, sealable bags and stack into the freezer to store until needed.
3. To cook, leave to thaw in the bag before emptying into a hot frying pan to sauté with veggies, rice, egg or whatever you fancy!

MARINATED PORK PACKETS

Slices of pork, marinated with simple herbs, olive oil, and lemon juice that can serve with a side of fresh veggies and roasted potatoes, or in pita bread with salad and Greek yoghurt.

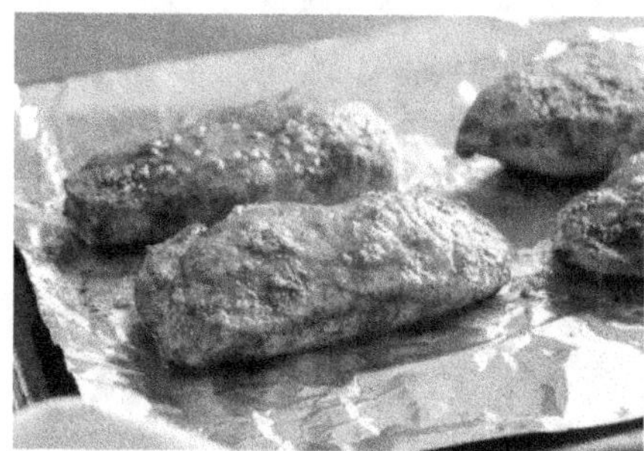

Serves: 8 packets, (1 serving per packet)

Container: you will need 8 freezer-friendly, sealable bags

Time: approximately 15 minutes

Nutritional info per serving:

- Calories: 220
- Fat: 39 grams
- Protein: 21 grams
- Carbs: 2 grams

Ingredients:

- 4 pork steaks, cut into slices
- 2 tbsp. olive oil
- Juice of 1 lemon
- 1 small sprig of fresh rosemary, roughly chopped
- 1 tsp. dried mixed herbs (use fresh herbs if you have them, but don't worry if you don't, dried herbs are fine)
- 4 garlic cloves, crushed

Method:

1. Place all the ingredients into a bowl and stir to combine, making sure the pork is thoroughly coated in oil, lemon juice, garlic and herbs.
2. Divide between 8 freezer-safe bags, seal and stack into the freezer to store until needed.
3. Leave to thaw before cooking in a hot frying pan.

PREPPED PASTA SAUCE: TOMATO

Keeping some frozen pasta sauces in the freezer is one of the best ways to utilize the magic of meal prepping. Boil some wholegrain or gluten-free pasta and throw one of these sauce packets into a pot to thaw and cook through. The first one in this series is a simple and tasty tomato sauce.

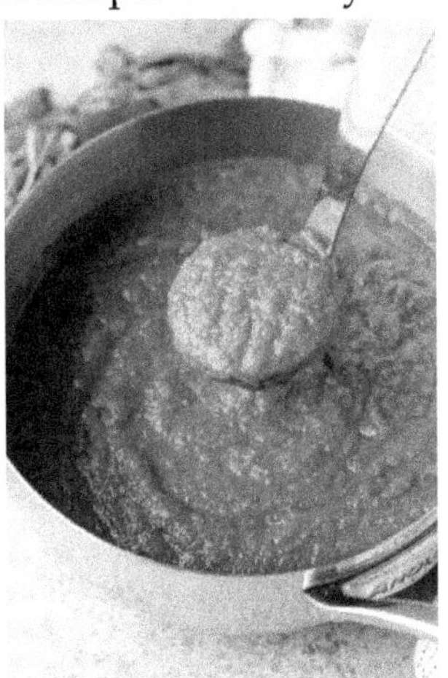

Serves: 4 containers of sauce (each container has enough sauce for 3 servings of pasta)

Container: you will need 4 airtight, freezer-friendly containers

Time: approximately 25 minutes

Nutritional info per serving:

- Calories: 55
- Fat: 3 grams
- Protein: 1 gram
- Carbs: 8 grams

Ingredients:

- Olive oil
- 6 garlic cloves, finely chopped
- 2 onions, finely chopped
- 3 cans (14 oz.) chopped tomatoes
- 2 tbsp. balsamic vinegar
- 1 tsp. honey
- 1 tsp. mixed dried herbs
- Salt and pepper, to taste

Method:

1. Drizzle the olive oil in a frying pan and heat it over medium heat.
2. Add the garlic and onions to the pan and sauté until soft.
3. Add the tomatoes, balsamic vinegar, honey, herbs, and a pinch of salt, and pepper, stir to combine.

4. Cover the pot and leave to simmer on a low heat for 20 minutes.
5. Leave the sauce to cool slightly before dividing between 4 containers, cover, and pack into the freezer to store until needed!
6. You could also use this sauce for zucchini noodles and meatballs!

PREPPED PASTA SAUCE: PESTO

This sauce is not for the freezer, but for the fridge. Spoon it into a glass jar or airtight container and place a dollop onto your zoodles or wholegrain pasta next time you're in a rush for the dinner. You don't need much of this pesto, as it has a strong and rich flavor. This is an ideal recipe for people who have lots of basil growing in their herb garden!

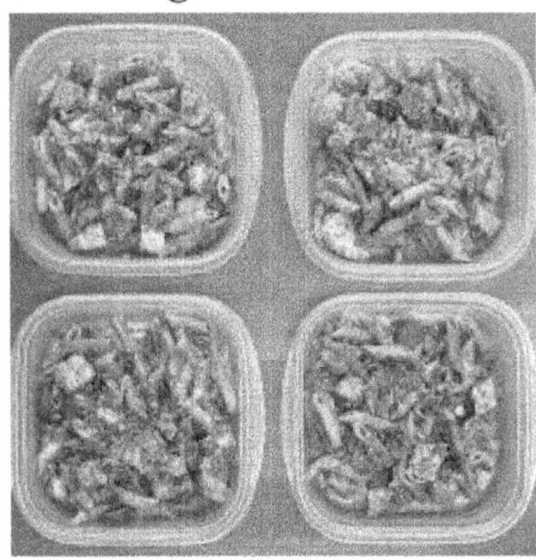

Serves: makes enough for about 12 servings

Container: you will need 1 glass jar with a lid, or a sealable container

Time: approximately 10 minutes

Nutritional info per serving:

- **Calories: 130**
- Fat: 12 grams
- Protein: 4 grams
- Carbs: 1 gram

Ingredients:

- 2 cups fresh basil leaves
- 3.5 oz. parmesan cheese, broken into small chunks
- 1/3 cup olive oil
- 3 garlic cloves, roughly chopped
- ½ cup pine nuts, (they are very expensive so just use cashew nuts for a cheaper option!)
- Salt and pepper, to taste

Method:

1. Place all the ingredients in a blender or small food processor and add a pinch of salt and pepper.
2. Blend until smooth but still with a few small pieces of nuts remaining.
3. Pour into your jar or container and store in the fridge until needed!

4. You can also use this as a salad dressing for potato salads or chicken salads.

PREPPED PASTA SAUCE: CREAMY MUSHROOM

The slightly lighter option of the traditional creamy sauce uses a part of sour cream and a part of yoghurt for a tangy flavor. This earthy mushroom sauce is lovely on pasta or zoodles, but it's also ideal when served on a grilled steak or chicken. Keep a few packets of this sauce in the freezer and throw straight into a pot over a medium heat when you want to use it!

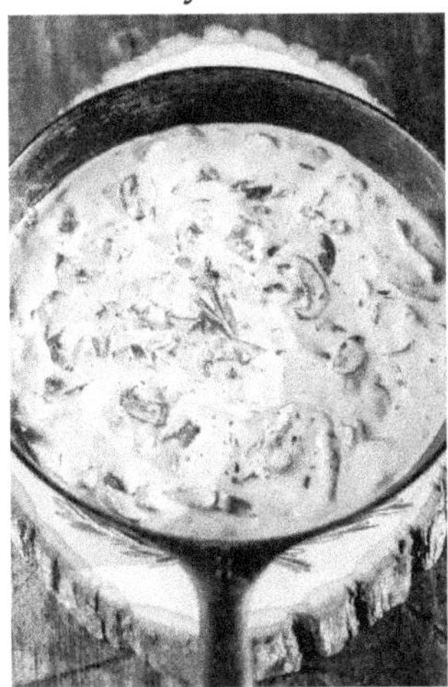

Serves: 4 containers of sauce (each container has enough for about 3 servings)

Container: you will need 4 airtight, freezer-safe containers

Time: approximately 20 minutes

Nutritional info per serving:

- Calories: 80
- Fat: 4 grams
- Protein: 2 grams
- Carbs: 3 grams

Ingredients:

- 2 tbsp. olive oil
- 5 cups chopped mushrooms (use a range of different kinds of mushrooms if you like! I use white button mushrooms and Portobello mushrooms)
- 8 garlic cloves, finely chopped
- 1 sprig of fresh rosemary, finely chopped
- 3fl oz. white wine
- ½ cup (4fl oz.) sour cream
- ½ cup (4fl oz.) plain yogurt

Method:

1. Drizzle the olive oil into a frying pan and heat over medium heat.

2. Add the mushrooms, garlic and rosemary or mixed herbs, sauté for a few minutes until the mushrooms have begun to shrink and become brownish.
3. Add the wine and simmer until the alcohol evaporates.
4. Add the sour cream and yoghurt and stir to combine.
5. Turn off the heat and leave the sauce to cool slightly before dividing between 4 containers, cover and place into the freezer to store until needed!

HEALTHY LAMB CURRY WITH COUSCOUS

Couscous is a tasty alternative to rice, and it goes so well with this tasty lamb curry. Tomatoes, spices, onions, and lamb cooked together to create a rich and aromatic curry to soak into a small bed of soft couscous. Great for the freezer!

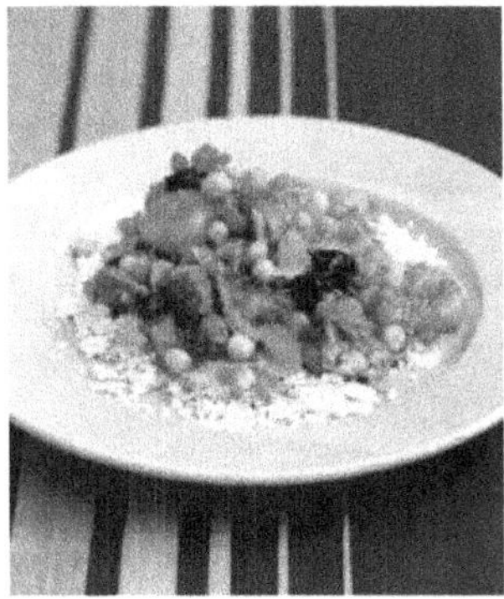

Serves: 6

Container: you will need 6 airtight containers

Time: approximately 30 minutes

Nutritional info per serving:

- Calories: 650
- Fat: 29 grams
- Protein: 43 grams
- Carbs: 52 grams

Ingredients:

- Olive oil
- 2 onions roughly chopped
- 1 tsp. ground turmeric
- 1 tsp. chili powder
- 1 tsp. dried cumin
- 1 tsp. dried coriander
- ½ tsp. cinnamon
- 20 oz. lamb steak (leg steak works great), cut into cubes
- 2 cups (16fl oz.) lamb stock
- 2 cans (14 oz.) chopped tomatoes
- Salt and pepper, to taste
- 2 cups dried couscous

Method:

1. Drizzle some olive oil in a large frying pan or pot and heat over a medium heat.
2. Add the onions, turmeric, chili powder, cumin, coriander, and cinnamon and heat until the onions are soft.

3. Add the lamb cubes and stir to coat in spices and onions, sauté for a couple of minutes to brown the meat.
4. Add the lamb stock, tomatoes, salt and pepper, stir to combine.
5. Place the lid onto the pot or pan and allow it to simmer over a low heat for about 25 minutes until the lamb is cooked and the curry sauce is rich and beginning to thicken.
6. While the curry cooks, prepare the couscous: place the dried couscous in a bowl and pour 2 and a half cups of boiling water over, cover the bowl and leave for about 5 minutes until the couscous is soft.
7. Uncover the couscous and add a pinch of salt and pepper, use a fork to fluff the couscous and then divide it between 6 containers.
8. Divide the lamb curry between the containers and spoon it on top of the couscous, cover and place into the fridge or freezer to store until needed!

SALMON WITH MANGO AND LENTILS

Treat yourself to a salmon dinner and make it a special one with mango and lentils. You can easily freeze this dish as salmon is preserved really well in the freezer. I like to make this dish when I feel like my body is calling out for some healthy fats and some fiber!

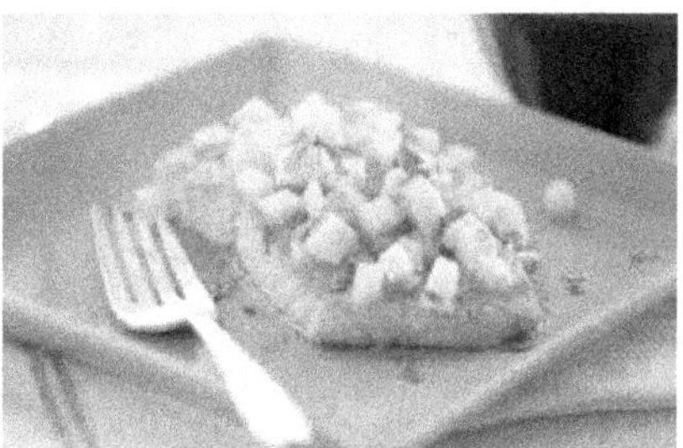

Serves: 4

Container: you will need 4 airtight containers

Time: approximately 20 minutes

Nutritional info per serving:

- Calories: 315
- Fat: 9 grams
- Protein: 30 grams
- Carbs: 26 grams

Ingredients:

- Olive oil
- 2 large salmon steaks, cut in half to make 4 even pieces
- 1 tbsp. soy sauce
- 1 tsp. sweet chili sauce
- 2 cups cooked brown lentils (I used canned ones, so much easier!)
- 1 ripe mango, skin removed, flesh cut into small chunks
- 4 fresh mint leaves, finely chopped

Method:

1. Drizzle some olive oil in a non-stick frying pan and heat it over medium heat.
2. Add the salmon pieces to the hot pan skin side down and cook for 2 minutes on each side or until just cooked through.
3. Pour the soy sauce and chili sauce over the salmon.
4. Divide the lentils between the 4 containers, add the mango to each container, then place a piece of salmon on top, finish by sprinkling each piece of salmon with the fresh mint.
5. Cover the containers and place into the fridge or freezer until needed!

FREEZER CHICKEN SOUP

This soup is an extremely light meal, filled with minerals and nutrients to restore you after a binge-full weekend. Chicken, broth, corn and scallions come together to melt into a tasty and wholesome soup to make you feel nourished.

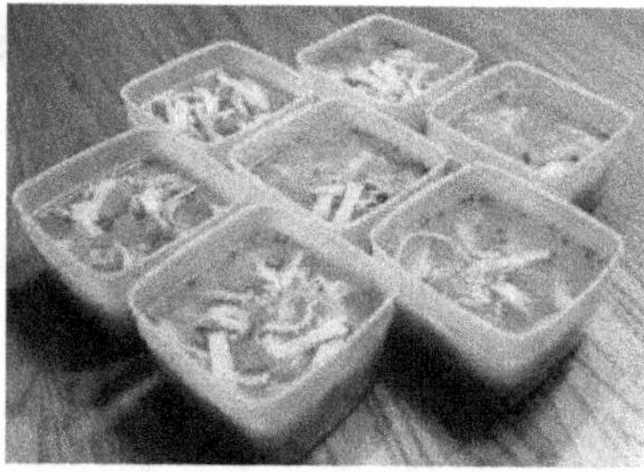

Serves: 6

Container: you will need 6 freezer-safe, airtight containers

Time: approximately 30 minutes

Nutritional info per serving:

- Calories: 230
- Fat: 9 grams
- Protein: 25 grams
- Carbs: 12 grams

Ingredients:

- 5 boneless chicken thighs, cut into small pieces
- 1 onion, finely chopped
- 4 cups (32fl oz.) chicken broth
- 2 cups (16fl oz.) water
- 1 can (14 oz.) corn kernels, drained
- 2 scallions, finely sliced
- Salt and pepper, to taste

Method:

1. Place all the ingredients in a pot and add a pinch of salt and pepper, heat over a medium heat and cover.
2. Leave to simmer for approximately 30 minutes until the chicken is cooked through.
3. Leave to cool slightly before dividing between 6 containers, cover and stack into the freezer to store until needed.
4. Leave the frozen containers on the counter to thaw before thoroughly reheating, or simply place the frozen soup in a pot over a high heat to speed the process up!

SNACKS AND DRESSINGS

When you feel like having something to chew on while working or dealing with house chores, we usually reach out for those unhealthy snacks and munches, bought in the store and packed with sugars and unhealthy carbs.

Thus, having some snacks in your fridge, on hand when you need something light and fast is always a good idea, and the next recipes will give you a strong hold on healthier snacks to keep your weight-loss goals going strong.

AUTHENTIC AVOCADO TOAST

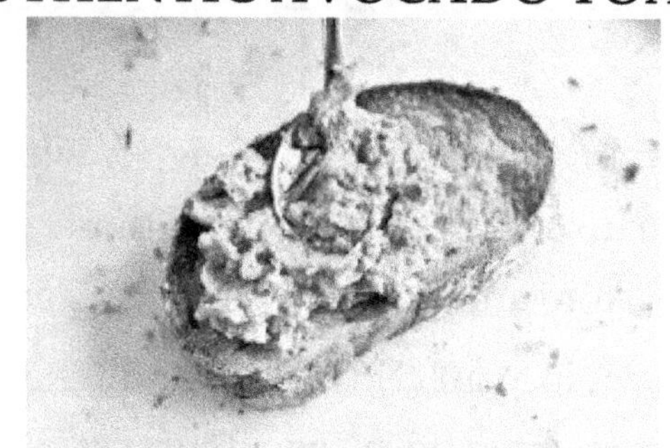

Prepping time: 10 minutes\ **Cooking time:** 3 minutes

Servings: 2

Container: 2 small containers

Ingredients:

- 4 slice of toasted whole wheat bread
- ½ ripe avocado
- Flaky sea salt
- Freshly cracked black pepper
- Flavorful olive oil
- Crushed red pepper flakes

Preparation:

- Slice the avocado and spread over the toast
- With a fork, mash the avocado slices
- Sprinkle with a bit of sea salt with a few grinds of black pepper
- Drizzle with olive oil and garnish with red pepper flakes
- Transfer to 2 small containers and store in the fridge for 2-3 days until needed.

Nutrition Values

- Protein: 7g
- Carbs: 28g
- Fats: 15g
- Calories: 250

THAI EDAMAME WITH SESAME SEEDS

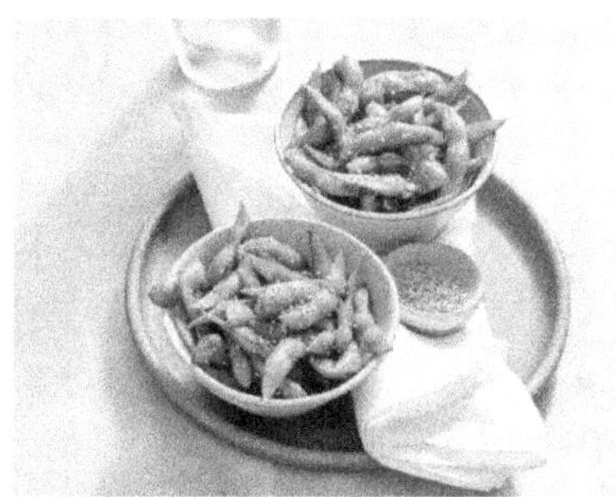

Prepping time: 10 minutes\ **Cooking time:** 3 minutes

Servings: 2

Container: 2 small containers

Ingredients:

- 3 tablespoons of water
- 4 cups of Edamame pods
- 2 tablespoons of light brown sugar
- 1 tablespoon of toasted sesame oil
- 1 tablespoon of rice vinegar
- ½ teaspoon of kosher salt
- ½ teaspoon of freshly ground black pepper
- 1 teaspoon of toasted sesame seeds

Preparation:

- In a large skillet over medium-high heat, bring the water to a boil
- Add Edamame pods and cover
- Let them cook for about 2 minutes
- Add oil, sugar, pepper, vinegar, and brown sugar
- Cook for another 2-3 minutes until the liquid has evaporated
- Make sure that the pods are fully coated
- Transfer Edamame pods to 2 serving containers and sprinkle with sesame seeds
- Store in the fridge for 2-3 days until needed.

Nutrition Values

- Protein: 3g
- Carbs: 7g
- Fats: 4g
- Calories: 73

SUBTLE ROASTED EGGPLANT WITH FETA DIP

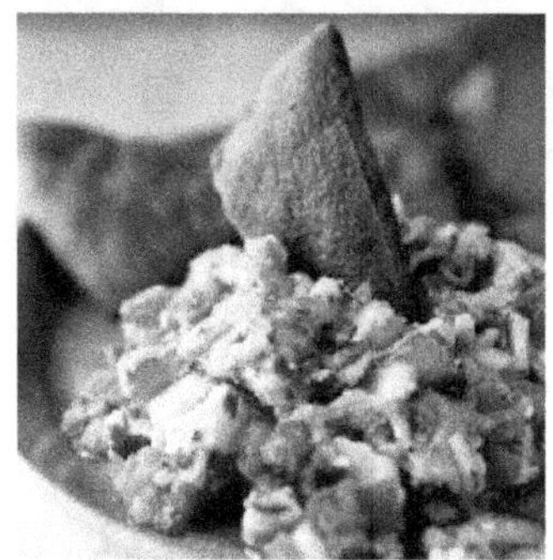

Prepping time: 20 minutes\ Cooking time: 20 minutes

Servings: 6

Container: 6 small containers

Ingredients:

- 1 medium eggplant
- 2 tablespoons of lemon juice
- ¼ cup of extra virgin olive oil
- ½ cup of crumbled feta cheese
- 1 finely chopped small red bell pepper
- 1 small seeded and minced chili pepper
- 2 tablespoons of chopped fresh basil
- 1 tablespoon of finely chopped flat-leaf parsley
- ¼ teaspoon of cayenne pepper
- ¼ teaspoon of salt
- Just a pinch of sugar

Preparation:

- Preheat the oven to 350 degrees Fahrenheit, positioning the oven rack about 6 inches from the heating element
- Line a baking pan with foil and place the eggplant in the pan
- Gently poke holes all over the eggplant using a fork
- Bake the eggplant for about 18 minutes, turning it every 5 minutes
- Transfer the charred eggplant to a cutting board and let it cool
- In a medium sized bowl, add lemon juice
- Cut the eggplant in half lengthwise and scoop the flesh into the bowl
- Toss the flesh with the juice
- Add some oil and mash the mixture using a fork
- Stir in onion, feta, chili pepper, bell pepper, parsley, basil, salt and cayenne

- Mix well
- Season with sugar if desired
- Transfer to 6 small containers and store in the fridge until needed.

Nutrition Values

- Protein: 2g
- Carbs: 4g
- Fats: 6g
- Calories: 76

MEAN AND GREEN FRITTERS

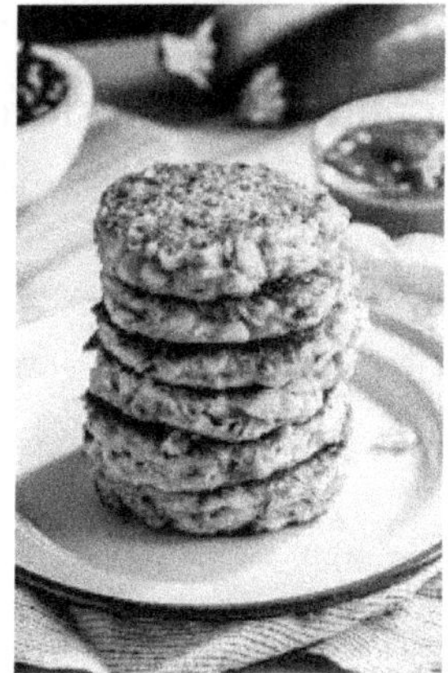

Prepping time: 15 minutes \ Cooking time: 15 minutes

Servings: 3

Container: 3 small containers

Ingredients:

- 5oz of grated courgettes
- 3 medium eggs
- 3oz of finely chopped broccoli florets
- Small package of roughly chopped dill
- 3 tablespoons of gluten-free flour
- 2 tablespoons of sunflower oil

Preparation:

- Squeeze the courgettes with your hands or twist in a towel to ensure that the moisture is removed
- Beat the eggs in a small bowl
- Add the broccoli, courgettes, and dill, reserving some dill for garnish
- Mix everything well
- Add the flour and season with salt and pepper
- Mix again
- In a medium sized frying pan, heat the oil over medium heat
- Use a large serving spoon to scoop the batter into the pan to make the the fritters
- Cook for 3-4 minutes until one side is browned
- Flip the fritters over and until the other side is cooked as well
- Keep repeating the process until all of the batter is used
- Divide the cooked fritters between the containers, garnish with dill and transfer to the fridge to store until needed.

Nutrition Values

- Calories: 359
- Fat: 21g
- Carbohydrates: 25g
- Protein: 16g

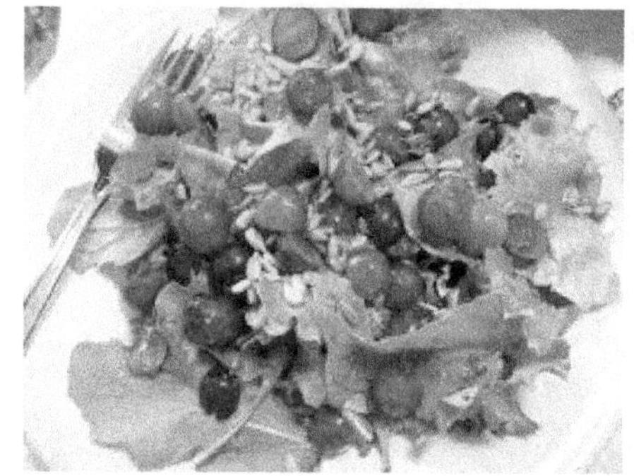

Prepping time: 10 minutes\ Cooking time: 0 minutes

Servings: 3

Container: 3 small containers

Ingredients:

- 3 tablespoons of red wine vinegar
- 1 teaspoon of honey
- 1 teaspoon of maple syrup
- ½ teaspoon of stone-ground mustard
- 2 teaspoons of rapeseed oil
- 7 cups of loosely packed baby arugula
- 2 cups of halved red grapes
- 2 tablespoons of toasted sunflower seeds
- 1 teaspoon of chopped fresh thyme
- ¼ teaspoon of salt
- ¼ teaspoon of freshly ground black pepper

Preparation:

- For the dressing, in a small bowl, whisk honey, vinegar, syrup, rapeseed oil, and mustard
- Place arugula in a salad bowl and add the seeds, thyme, and grapes mix to combine
- Drizzle with dressing
- Season with pepper and salt
- Toss and divide between the containers before transferring to the fridge and storing until needed!

Nutrition Values

- Calories: 81
- Fat: 31g
- Carbohydrates: 13g
- Protein: 16g

BOWL OF RICOTTA AND TOASTED ALMONDS!

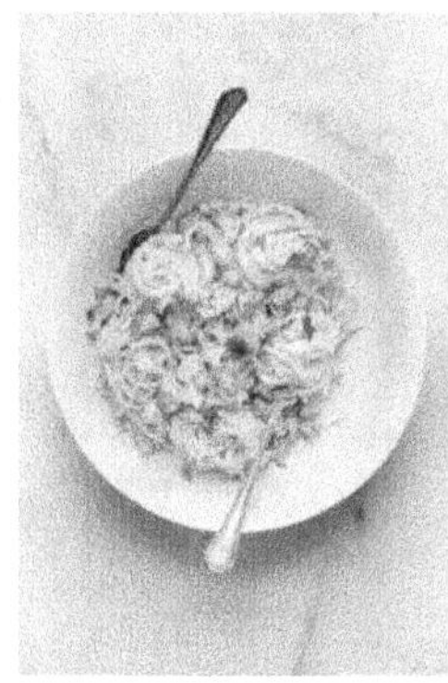

Prepping time: 10 minutes\ Cooking time: 0 minutes

Servings: 2

Container: 2 small containers

Ingredients:

- ¾ cup of frozen and pitted cherries
- 2 tablespoons of part-skimmed ricotta
- 1 tablespoon of toasted silvered almonds
- 2 teaspoons olive oil
- 1 tablespoon of freshly-squeezed lemon juice

Preparation:

- Microwave the cherries for 1-2 minutes or until they are warmed through
- Top with ricotta and almonds.
- Drizzle the olive oil and lemon juice and stir to combine
- Divide between containers and store in the fridge until needed.

Nutrition Values

- Calories: 155
- Fat: 6g
- Carbohydrates: 22g
- Protein: 6

GORGEOUSLY SWEET OVEN-FRIED POTATOES

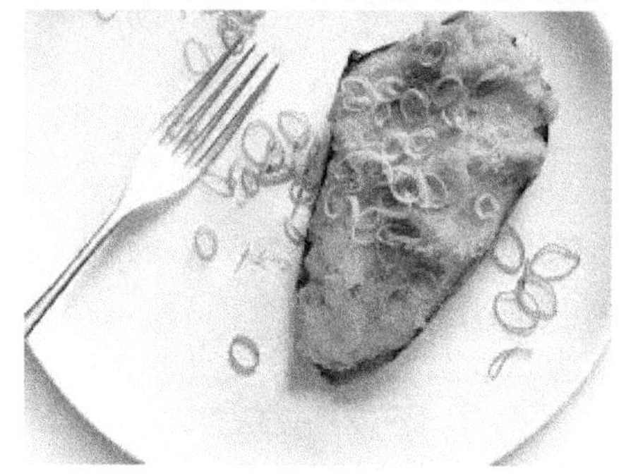

Prepping time: 10 minutes\ **Cooking time:** 30 minutes

Servings: 2

Container: 2 medium containers

Ingredients:

- 2 medium potatoes, cut into thick slices
- ¼ teaspoon of pepper
- Vegetable cooking spray
- 1 tablespoon of finely chopped fresh parsley
- 1 teaspoon of grated orange rind
- 1 minced garlic clove

Preparation:

- Preheat the oven to 400 degrees Fahrenheit
- Coat a baking sheet with cooking spray
- Arrange the potatoes in a single layer on the baking sheet
- Bake the potatoes for about 30 minutes
- Turn the potatoes halfway through
- In a small bowl, mix the pepper, parsley, orange rind, and garlic
- Transfer the potatoes to your containers.
- Sprinkle the seasoning over baked potato slices; cover the containers and store in the fridge until needed.

Nutrition Values

- Calories: 178
- Fat: 25g
- Carbohydrates: 366g
- Protein: 25g

SOFTEST AND JUICIEST COCONUT BANANAS

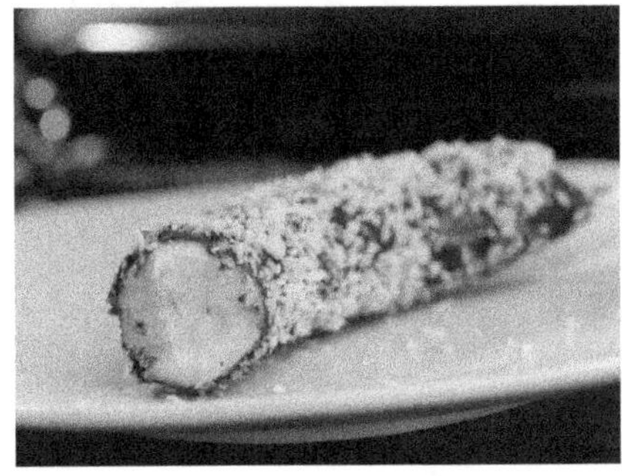

Prepping time: 10 minutes\ Cooking time: 0 minutes

Servings: 2

Container: 2 small containers or 1 medium container

Ingredients:

- 4 teaspoons of cocoa powder
- 4 teaspoons of toasted unsweetened coconut
- 2 sliced small bananas

Preparation:

- Add the cocoa powder to one plate and toasted coconut on another
- Roll the banana slices first in the cocoa followed by the toasted coconut
- Shake off any excess and transfer to the containers to store in the fridge until needed!

Nutrition Values

- Protein: 1g
- Carbs: 13g
- Fats: 1g
- Calories: 6

ENERGIZING BALLS OF PEANUT AND OAT

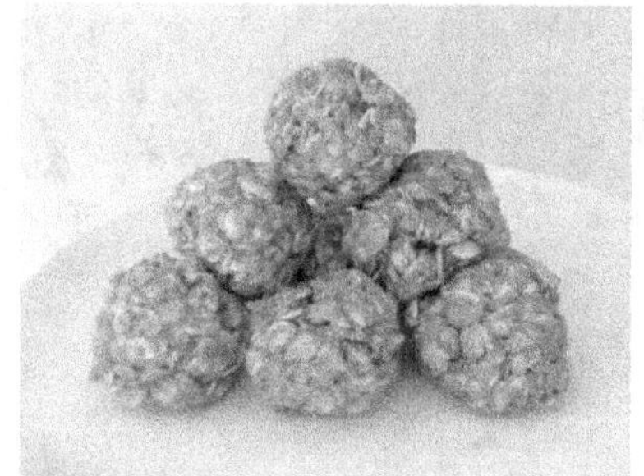

Prepping time: 15 minutes \ **Cooking time:** 15 minutes

Servings: makes 12 balls

Container: 1 medium container

Ingredients:

- ¾ cup of chopped up Medjool dates
- ½ cup of rolled oats
- ¼ cup of natural peanut butter
- Chia seeds as needed

Preparation:

- Soak the dates in hot water for about 10 minutes
- Drain the dates
- In a food processor, add oats, dates, and peanut butter and process well
- Roll the mixture into 12 balls
- Garnish the balls with chia seeds and transfer to your container.
- Chill the balls in your fridge and serve when needed!

Nutrition Values

- Protein: 2g
- Carbs: 73g
- Fats: 3g
- Calories: 73

CONCLUSION

Once you get the hang of meal prepping, you will never want to go back! Having packets of fresh, healthy food packed away in the fridge and freezer, ready to be eaten is a satisfying and gratifying feeling. If these recipes do not quite fit in with your particular weight-loss diet, then simply modify them until the macronutrients are where you want them to be! Less carbs? No worries. More protein? Easy. Just download a calorie-counting app, load the recipes in, and shuffle things around to reach your desired numbers.

Always remember to prep meals that you want to eat! In my opinion, the best foods are healthy and delicious, and once you hit that sweet-spot you can lose weight without even noticing that you've changed your diet! You'll be so satisfied and full from your yummy, nutrient-filled foods that you won't get that horrible sense of deprivation and craving which comes with many strict diets.

Make a day of it and go shopping for containers, oils, spices, non-perishables, masking tape and sharpies for labeling, a diary to plan your meals and prep days, and put it all in a pretty and space-saving box.

Make your prep-sessions fun and relaxing, as they should be! You deserve to enjoy your life, your diet, and your kitchen.

Good luck and have fun!

Legal & Disclaimer

The information contained in this book and its contents is not designed to replace or take the place of any form of medical or professional advice; and is not meant to replace the need for independent medical, financial, legal or other professional advice or services, as may be required. The content and information in this book has been provided for educational and entertainment purposes only.

The content and information contained in this book has been compiled from sources deemed reliable, and it is accurate to the best of the Author's knowledge, information and belief. However, the Author cannot guarantee its accuracy and validity and cannot be held liable for any errors and/or omissions. Further, changes are periodically made to this book as and when needed. Where appropriate and/or necessary, you must consult a professional (including but not limited to your doctor, attorney, financial advisor or such other professional advisor) before using any of the suggested remedies, techniques, or information in this book.

Upon using the contents and information contained in this book, you agree to hold harmless the Author from and against any damages, costs, and expenses, including any legal fees potentially resulting from the application of any of the information provided by this book. This disclaimer applies to any loss, damages or injury caused by the use and application, whether directly or indirectly, of any advice or information presented, whether for breach of contract, tort, negligence, personal injury, criminal intent, or under any other cause of action.

You agree to accept all risks of using the information presented inside this book.

You agree that by continuing to read this book, where appropriate and/or necessary, you shall consult a professional (including but not limited to your doctor, attorney, or financial advisor or such other advisor as needed) before using any of the suggested remedies, techniques, or information in this book.

Your Gift

I wanted to show my appreciation that you support my work so I've put together a free gift for you.

http://bonusfreebook.org/

Just visit the link above to download it now.

I know you will love this gift.

If you like this book, you can see and buy my other books on this link:

https://www.amazon.com/Lisa-Brook/e/B079TZXP62/ref=sr_ntt_srch_lnk_4?qid=1518768684&sr=1-4

Thank you for attention!

With love,

Lisa Brook